Justice and the
Human Genome Project

Justice and the Human Genome Project

TIMOTHY F. MURPHY AND
MARC A. LAPPÉ, EDITORS

UNIVERSITY OF CALIFORNIA PRESS
Berkeley   Los Angeles   London

University of California Press
Berkeley and Los Angeles, California

University of California Press
London, England

Library of Congress Cataloging-in-Publication Data

Justice and the human genome project / Timothy F. Murphy and Marc A. Lappé, editors.
    p.   cm.
Includes bibliographical references and index.
ISBN 0-520-08363-6 (acid-free paper)
1. Human gene mapping—Moral and ethical aspects—Congresses.
2. Human Genome Project—Congresses.   I. Murphy, Timothy F., 1954–.
II. Lappé, Marc.
QH445.2.J87   1994
174'.25—dc20
        93-18094
        CIP

Printed in the United States of America

1   2   3   4   5   6   7   8   9

The paper used in this publication meets the minimum requirements of American National Standard for Information Sciences—Permanence of Paper for Printed Library Materials, ANSI Z39.48-1984 ⊗

Contents

Preface

Timothy F. Murphy and Marc A. Lappé

The essays gathered in this volume were among those presented at a conference titled "Justice and the Human Genome" held in Chicago in early November 1991. The goal of that conference, sponsored by the U.S. Department of Energy and the University of Illinois at Chicago, was to consider questions of justice as they are and will be raised by the human genome project, that ambitious multinational effort to map and sequence the entire human genome. To achieve its goal of identifying and elucidating the challenges of justice inherent in genomic research and its social applications, the conference drew together in one forum members from academia, medicine, and industry in order to sketch out central questions that will follow the emergence of genomic profiling capabilities.

The essays in this volume address theoretical and practical concerns relative to the meaning of genomic research. Whether the authors are concerned with the history of eugenics, the meaning of individual differences, or access to health care, they are all united in their concern about the impact of genomic research on individual persons and their place in specific ethnic and cultural groups. If there is a common goal underlying the analyses here, it is the protection of individual persons and cultural groups from unjust social prejudices and arrangements that would burden individual choice or degrade the worth of certain groups defined in invidious ways. It is perhaps a measure of the age that we express as much anxiety as hope with regards to the human genome project. It is the goal of this volume to resist inappropriate anxiety by offering moral analysis that resists facile and corrupting uses of genomic research but that nevertheless emphasizes the very real significance and importance of genomic research.

While many of the concerns raised about the genome project have a fantastic quality to them, Timothy F. Murphy, in "The Genome Project and the Meaning of Difference," nevertheless cautions against certain subtle effects of a coordinated scientific project whose goal is a characterization of the human genome. By reason of the conforming forces involved in carrying out a centrally coordinated program of research and the inevitable influence of a "standard" human genome in biomedical thinking, genomic research may have the effect of working against incentives to scientific progress and tolerance of human diversity. In a cautionary vein, he notes this paradox of science: even as it advances the realm of human knowledge and offers ways to alleviate human suffering, it may have the effect of foreclosing avenues of scientific novelty and of raising barriers to acceptance of moral and human diversity.

Perhaps part of the special moral concern that has been expressed about genomic research belongs to the decidedly problematic history of eugenics movements. In "Eugenics and the Human Genome Project: Is the Past Prologue?" Daniel J. Kevles addresses this concern, noting the way in which eugenics movements in American and world history have been linked to intolerable moral judgments about the worth and worthlessness of individuals. Despite the many dark moments in the history of eugenics, Kevles does not see that the current genome project is vulnerable to the kind of tendentious distinctions drawn by eugenicists in the past because of the democratic nature of our social institutions, because there are now powerful antieugenic constituencies, because we now better understand that desirable and complex human traits are not amenable to simple-minded genetic interventions, and because we now better appreciate the horrors of past eugenic brutalities.

Arthur L. Caplan, in "Handle with Care: Race, Class, and Genetics," likewise notes the way in which the future of genomic studies is often discussed in terms of the villainy of recent genetic history and politics. But, he argues, genomic research need not fall victim to the prejudicial ideologies of the past, especially if public debate protects people whose social circumstances may be made vulnerable by genomic studies. In a kind of thought experiment, Caplan outlines certain scenarios that might occur in the future, scenarios that point out ways in which genomic profiling can generate dilemmas about identity, affirmative action, privacy, immigration, and reproductive choices. It becomes clear that the history of genetic study may not confine genomic research, but neither will genomic research be free of troubling social choices as to its fair and equitable use.

In "Public Choices and Private Choices: Legal Regulation of Genetic Testing," Lori B. Andrews reviews certain legal and policy precedents that frame the context in which decisions about genetic testing will be made in the future. She pays special attention to genetic testing in reproduction, noting ways in which the law either permits, forbids, or requires certain forms of reproductive testing and choices and also noting the ways in which individual desires may conflict with social objectives. She concludes this review by observing that genetic testing may well threaten, as other forces have, that traditional and comfortable distinction we have long drawn between the private and the public.

Looking at an idea that has a central importance in American political and social thought, in "Rules for Gene Banks: Protecting Privacy in the Genetics Age," George J. Annas considers the implications of "gene banks" for privacy. Gene banks would ostensibly store genetic samples or genomic profiles of individuals, and Annas proposes that certain respected liberties can only be maintained in the age of gene banking through considered and swift deliberation of rules governing the collection and storage of genetic materials. Toward that end, he proposes certain rules for consideration, rules that require public notice of the establishment of gene banks, informed consent in their policies, and restricted use of their samples.

Robert J. Pokorski, in "Uses of Genetic Information by Private Insurers," identifies an issue of genomic research that is of central concern to the insurance industry: access to the genomic profiling of individuals that genome research is expected to make possible. The use of genomic profiling is of special concern to a society in which the burdens of health care (and life insurance) are left to individual resources and employers. Although there may be a fear that genomic profiling will be used prejudicially against people at risk of genetic disease, Pokorski argues that insurers need access to such information to set insurance costs according to the actual degree of risk that belongs to given individuals. Access to genomic profiling will preserve the principle of equity that Pokorski thinks essential to the ability of insurers to protect not only their own solvency but also their continued ability to provide insurance benefits in ways that do not unjustly burden people less at risk of genetic disadvantages.

In contrast to this position, Norman Daniels raises an important

philosophical question by asking to what extent it is fair to let people
benefit from personal advantages when those advantages have their
origin in a random genetic distribution. One's genetic predisposition
to disease or health, after all, is a matter of biological accident. It is
for this reason that Daniels prefers to emphasize the significance of
"adverse selection" not as a matter of securing coverage at rates disproportionately unprofitable for insurers but as a matter of extending
coverage at disproportionately profitable rates. Daniels then argues
that the standards of equity inherent in current insurance programs
violate certain moral standards and do not protect equality of opportunity in health. He therefore rejects the view that health advantages or disadvantages should be treated like mere economic assets
and argues instead for a view that requires the protection of health
in ways independent of its genetic origin. He also notes some implications of genomic research for public understandings of the nature
of responsibility for health, especially since genomic research may
elicit either fatalism or hypercaution as regards the relationship between genes and health.

In "Just Genetics: A Problem Agenda," Leonard M. Fleck addresses the matter of emerging genetic technologies that may both
eliminate genetic disabilities and enhance genetic superiority. While
he rightly argues that there is sometimes an unclear line between
what constitutes disability and enhancement, he nevertheless thinks
that genetic technologies that aim at the elimination of clear genetic
deficits ought to have moral priority over other biomedical interventions. Fleck thinks that from a disinterested point of view, people
would assign priority to the development of genetic technologies over
other biomedical technologies—such as artificial hearts—since genetic disabilities end in profound disabilities and premature death
for which there are no other means of avoidance, social remedy, or
recompense. Moreover, such a priority would also respect the principle of arranging social benefits to favor those who are least well off.

In the essay closing the volume, Marc Lappé points out ways in
which genomic research will raise and sharpen questions of social
equity not only with regards to screening and employment but also
to questions of compensation. Genomic profiling can be expected to
establish differences not only among individuals but also among
groups, thereby raising questions of social equity in the way we value
and disvalue heritable traits. He notes, too, ways in which genomic

differences may extend questions of moral equity to domains we at present believe belong to accidents of nature.

All the essays raise issues that are likely to continue as matters of debate and concern even as we advance further and further into the genomic era. Part of what makes this volume unique is what has made the human genome project unique from its inception: its consideration of the ethical, legal, and social implications of genomic research *before* that research has completed its tasks and *before* genomic applications have begun to alter social and institutional arrangements and policies. The human genome project will be no secretive Manhattan Project whose hidden research ultimately changed the political fate of the world forever and whose influences are still being measured to this day. The human genome project is by design self-conscious: its design anticipates and subjects the future to deliberation. This kind of planned moral and social deliberation—and the funding it was given—is without precedent in the history of scientific research. These essays must not be seen, then, as only a contribution to the ethical, legal, and social studies of the genome project. These essays are also themselves part of a grand experiment in attempting to assess in advance the significance of scientific research for the moral and political concepts by which we define ourselves. The challenge of these essays is thus twofold: to illuminate the genome project itself and to justify the hope placed in a study of this kind so that science and society can go forward in equitable relations. It is in the spirit of this challenge that we offer the essays that follow.

1

THE GENOME PROJECT AND THE MEANING OF DIFFERENCE

Timothy F. Murphy

In many ways, the current project to map and sequence the human genome appears to be that very kind of encyclopedic enterprise that Francis Bacon recommended in 1620 as part of his proposed "Great Instauration" of science.[1] Against a science he saw mired in and confounded by philosophical speculation, Bacon advocated a painstaking study of the material—not the metaphysical—properties of the world. He thus recommended exhaustive accounts of rainbows, frost, floods, birds, sleep, dreams, drugs, baking, bodily growth, medicine, wine, and so on for page after page. Given the magnitude of the studies he foresaw, it is not surprising that Bacon, Lord Chancellor under James I and VI, pleaded for state funding of research, thereby giving him the distinction of being the "father" of the federal research grant. He thought the costs of the "natural histories" he proposed would be well justified because they would lead to human power over the world, a world in which human interests were freed from the vicissitudes of fate and protected and promoted by human knowledge.[2] The goal of human study, he said, was "the knowledge of causes, and secret motions of things; and the enlarging of the bounds of human empire, to the effecting of all things possible."[3] And a society devoted to these pursuits would be, in the end, a "New Atlantis."

The human genome project appears to be a Baconian enterprise ("big science" we call it today), not only in its ambitions, its enormous costs, and the necessary involvement of government but also in its capacity to offer knowledge about the secret motion of things biological. There are questions, of course, about whether this initia-

1

tive will or should lead to the effecting of all things possible, and there are also questions about whether these ambitions, costs, and outcomes will advance our own society toward its New Atlantis. The New Atlantis described by Bacon, after all, was a harmonious, homogeneous utopia protected from the strife of the world by its remote distance from world events. It was a society dedicated to a single religion. Our own society, in contrast, is in many ways at the mercy of events wherever they might occur in the world. It is also a society deeply marked and divided by religion, race, economics, natural resources, culture, politics, and disease.

There is already a growing body of moral analysis that has attempted to characterize the quandaries and challenges of the genome project, and this analysis has raised many of the relevant questions even if it has not been able to offer definitive answers. Some of this analysis has been at pains to point out undesirable consequences of possible uses of genomic data, especially in discriminatory social practices. While it is important to be aware of these outcomes, it seems to me that what moral philosophy can also profitably contribute to the discussion is something other than prophesies of possible objectionable use of genomic characterizations. Health care workers, insurance analysts, attorneys, and other involved parties are often better situated than philosophers to predict unhappy consequences of the genome project. What philosophers can contribute seems to lie in another vein: interpreting the meaning of the project and its uses. I therefore want to identify here some of what I consider to be the main moral problematics of the genome project itself, issues that have to do with the nature and consequences of our commitment to this project. I also want to consider the genome project insofar as it raises philosophical questions about the nature and meaning of *difference.* This is a difficult task and one that is only begun here, but it is one that attempts, first, to get at the question of what it means to be engaged in a project to map and sequence the human genome and to ask, second, in what ways the genome project will work for or against human difference and alter the way in which we understand the worth of the individual in relationship to the social order.

MORAL ASPECTS OF THE GENOME PROJECT

Alexander M. Capron has observed that the genome project itself has proved of little ethical interest: "My personal sense is that persons assigned to discuss the ethics of genome mapping quickly find themselves discussing related subjects, because the topic-in-chief is regarded as pretty thin gruel."[4] Like most analysts, Capron therefore underlines the importance of analyzing the *uses* of the information the genome project is expected to generate.[5] In particular, in an *Emory Law Journal* article, he expresses concern about ownership and control over knowledge generated by the project. Capron is surely right in noting the way in which commentators have shied away from discussing "the topic-in-chief." Indeed, most ethical analysis of the genome project typically shies away from any suggestion that the project itself is morally problematic.

But is it true that there is little or no moral substance in the genome project itself? I think such a conclusion should be resisted; on the contrary, there are some important moral problematics to be considered. There are, first of all, questions about whether this venture is something that a society ought to undertake given other pressing needs. To what extent, after all, should a society undertake a project whose beneficiaries, in the main, exist in the future? James D. Watson and Robert Mullan Cook-Deegan have said that the primary objective of the human genome project is to aid in the assault on disease.[6] But that assault will not, for the most part, benefit living people, and a financial commitment of the kind involved in the genome project may mean that care will not be offered to actually existing people who here and now suffer from various diseases or natural or social ills. While it may be wise to prepare a future in which genetic diseases do not cause the damage they do now, it is not clear that there is anything but a supererogatory duty to do so. Thus, the question of the genome project may be put into relief this way: what is the moral argument to be offered that the suffering of people here and now can be sacrificed to expected benefits in the future?

In this vein, it is also worth considering whether and to what extent the genome project may amount to an evasion of contemporary social and medical problems, problems that we could address and possibly overcome if only we so chose. Should we, after all, be trying to develop methods to identify and eradicate genetically defective individuals through prenatal and neonatal genetic testing (and possibly abortion) rather than undertaking social accommodation of genetically disadvantaged people, finding what ways we can to offer them hope and happiness? Of course, there would be no relief for some of the genetically disadvantaged, but it is still worth wondering to what extent the living have priority over the future-living.

Even if there are possible answers to these questions, still the genome project may be problematic from another quarter. The genome project is "big science" and even bigger consequences are expected from it, but insofar as the project represents a coordinated plan of study, the potential exists for its functioning as a scientific and moral ideology because it is committed to a single way of representing genetic information and carrying with it the seeds of its own moral authority. The genome project, therefore, has the potential of functioning as an ideology with all the undesirable effects of ideology in conforming people and their expectations.[7]

Although there have been other government-sponsored programs of scientific study before it, the human genome project has special moral significance insofar as it may suggest a precedent that future scientific study is properly a matter of large-scale, federally financed, centrally coordinated projects. It is not wrong, of course, that the government should undertake such projects of scientific study; the question is whether this kind of undertaking is the best way for science and scientists to proceed. With its economic supports, the federal government has in effect created a scientific orthodoxy, and it is worth wondering whether this approach will have the effect of counterproductively suppressing the element of novelty so important to scientific advance. It is important to keep in mind, after all, that every time there are converts to a scientific project, voices of dissent capable of correcting and advancing human knowledge and wisdom may be lost.[8]

But perhaps these questions do not seem essential or significant as matters relevant to the genome project itself. Maybe they are not, but perhaps there is another explanation of why these questions have not been raised with special urgency. Perhaps it is because we commentators and analysts of the genome project already share common answers to such questions; our assumptions in common belie deep divisions of opinion. Perhaps there is no dwelling on moral aspects of the genome project per se because there are no disputants to conduct a debate about the project, this because the nation's intelligentsia has almost to a person already and predictably come down on the side of the project. In an age entirely comfortable with the promises and priorities of science, we do not have the sense that science (in contrast to its uses) is morally problematic. Except for research that may jeopardize people without their consent, we seem to have lost the sense that there can be research that "goes too far." We seem to have adopted as our own that single internal imperative of science: to know everything. We are prepared to wait until after the work of science is done to deal with any unhappy consequences it may make possible, and we have faith that our social institutions can absorb limitless advances in biomedical, physical, and social science. Therefore, far from being without moral interest, it seems to me that the genome project is remarkable as evidence of our collective and uniform moral and scientific expectations.

There is no reason, of course, why serious arguments against the genome project could not be raised on grounds of resource allocation, scientific openness, limits of inquiry, and possibly religious reasons as well. That they have not says more about us as a society than it does about the nature of the genome project itself. That there is no chorus of voices raised against the genome project per se does not mean that the project is itself without moral significance. The silence here is more likely the result of our society's homogeneous views as regards the morality of scientific inquiry in general or perhaps the result of the erroneous view that scientific inquiry is itself value free and only morally significant with regards to its consequences. Given approximately equivalent educational opportunities and social ideals, we perforce share common moral views, which is to say that our moral assumptions and conclusions can be hidden by the very virtue of their pervasive nature. I am *not* suggesting that we object to the genome project for the kinds of reasons raised here; I am merely observing that what passes as a question without moral significance may simply represent pervasive moral consensus. It is different views, different interpretations, different observers that make moral values obvious and open to debate.

It is evident, therefore, that at least one major meaning of the human genome project is that we as a society continue our commitment to academically orthodox science. We continue to place our hopes for the production of knowledge, and the economic and health opportunities it will make possible, in the hands of federally sponsored scientific researchers even to the extent that we cannot foresee the extent to which such knowledge will affect our social institutions and mores. We continue to have fairly unlimited optimism about the beneficence of science, this despite all the objectionable episodes that have occurred in research and in spite of the problems scientific research generates in its uses. We continue, in other words, to draw a clear distinction between science and its sins.

MARKING AND INTERPRETING DIFFERENCE

Beyond the moral significance of the project itself, the human genome project does indeed raise many interesting individual moral questions, questions related to the use of the tests and information it will produce. For example, it will be necessary to consider the ways in which resultant genetic probes should be used in matters of employment, insurability, money lending, reproduction, counseling, and so on. Genetic characterizations will also create a new class of health costs, and the question of how these costs will be met and ranked in the nation's social priorities will need to be addressed. There will also be questions of how experimentation in correcting genetic defects should be carried out and with what priority. Perplexing questions of equitable access and informed consent in such therapies will arise.

One of the major expectations of the genome project is that its information will offer people better health. But genetic characterizations are one thing and successful medical interventions to correct genetic dysfunctions are another. It is likely that there will be considerable lag time between the identification of genetic dysfunctions and interventions that can successfully alter them. It is also unclear at the present time whether widespread use of genetic characterizations (and possible treatments) will significantly improve the health of a nation's population. After all, we already know what it would take to improve the health of a considerable portion of the nation's population; it is just that we ignore the counsels against smoking, alcohol, failure to exercise, and so on.[9] Moreover, the use of genetic characterizations will not necessarily modify the course of the most socially significant diseases, such as communicable diseases. They may prove useful, on the contrary, for fairly rare occurrences that will not significantly alter the general distribution of nongenetic disease or the costs associated with such disease. These questions all deserve considerable attention as we shape policies and practices around genomic data.

But such questions do not themselves directly get at an underlying question that, in my mind, haunts the genome project. The ancient art of haruspicy attempted to divine the future through the examination of animal entrails. In our own time, are we now trying to foretell the future through the examination of "genetic entrails"? Certainly, we hope at least to be able to foretell the genetic future of particular individuals. Such a hope raises important questions regarding identity and difference. To what extent will the genome project generate new classes of human inferiority? Will the genome project generate a theoretical subjugation of genetically atypical people, born and unborn, and thereby establish difference as disease or disability? Will the genome project mark difference as an undesirable trait and justify its eradication?

The goal of the genome project is to produce a characterization of the human genetic complement in the way that anatomy produces a representation of the structural components of the human body or in the way that physiology represents bodily function. Thus, this genomic characterization will not identify the genome of a single person any more than anatomical or skeletal characterizations represent a given individual. Nevertheless, the genome project will offer a model by which to understand the functioning of genes and their relationships to particular organismal traits. And it is the existence of this model that lays the foundation for the interpretation of desirable and undesirable traits. The moral significance of the project may prove, therefore, to lie in its significance for the interpretation of health and disease, normalcy and difference.

There are many ways to represent the nature of human beings, and none of them are value neutral. Even a genomic characterization is already always determined by our social and conceptual background. What we see, therefore, in a genomic characterization of human beings depends on what we are accustomed to and interested in seeing, this for both the species as a whole and an individual in particular. There is no escaping this immersion in the social and conceptual preconditions of observation, representation, science, and language; we cannot ever hope to achieve the position of an entirely unconditioned, uninterested observer. Therefore, the moral question at issue here is not whether we can produce a value-neutral representation of human genetics but whether we can protect people from invidious interpretations of the representation that the genome project will offer.

There are many reasons to be cautious here. German philosopher Friedrich Nietzsche once observed, *"What one knows of oneself*—As soon as one animal sees another it measures itself against it in its mind, and men in barbarous ages did likewise. From this it follows that every man comes to know himself almost solely in regard to his powers of defence."[10] Coming as it does from a philosopher who was acutely aware of the importance of individuality and difference, this observation might even be interpreted to mean that marking differences *in order to assert and establish superiority* is even the primal form of thought itself. And history shows that difference is often the pretext for vilification and destruction of those marked in ways others are not.

It seems to me, therefore, that if there is a central moral issue at stake in the genome project, it is whether its characterizations will permit the erosion of difference in favor of genetic uniformity, whether its characterizations will offer yet another standard of "normalcy" to be used as a justification for the extermination of difference. It is in this regard that one needs to see and consider the nature of genome mapping. Will we, in finding new ways to mark the differences between people, invite new theories of personal and social worth, theories that presuppose standards of superiority and inferiority? There are already differences enough between people that are used as pretexts for their subjugation and villification. Will the genome project enlarge the power we already have in that regard?

Given their relative accessibility, the genetic characterization of newborns and fetuses would be one of the most likely venues for the identification and extinguishing of genetic defect or difference. It is perhaps worth recalling that it was not just National Socialist Germany alone that has had its own significant eugenics history.[11] Prior to World War II, the United States had its own very healthy eugenics movement. In advancing the cause of birth control, Margaret Sanger freely availed herself of language that bespeaks eugenic goals. She constantly spoke of the great number of children who should never have been born, those children who will pollute the race and drain the world of its resources.[12] If there was a central task facing the nation, Sanger thought it was the task of breeding a better race: "The noblest and most difficult art of all is the raising of human thoroughbreds." Accomplishing that goal required preventing the mass birth of inferior populations who were, in her view, responsible for the "ever-widening margins of biological waste." The goal should thus be to resist "the ever-increasing, unceasingly spawning classes of human beings who never should have been born at all," in which category she puts those whom she calls variously feeble sows' ears, the mentally and physically defective, degenerate stock, morons, the dregs of the human species, the blind, the deaf-mute, the degenerate, the nervous, the vicious, the idiotic, the imbecilic, the cretins, the epileptics, the feeble-minded, and in general the dead weight of human waste.

After the defeat of National Socialist Germany, the formal eugenics movement collapsed almost without a trace in the United States. But concern about defective children and adults lingers on in a different form. Whereas the eugenics movement offered its counsels in the language of preserving the race and husbanding resources, concern about the lives of the defective today is offered primarily in the language of "the best interests of the child." Fetuses are aborted and certain newborns are allowed to die, according to those making the decisions, because that course of action is in their "best interest." Moreover, defective children who survive are sometimes said to be the victims of "wrongful birth" or even "wrongful life."

Of course, genetic characterizations cannot predict with complete certainty which children will and will not express genetic disease, this because of the roles human variability and environmental differences play in the expression of disease. Genetic characterizations will, however, highlight *possible* differences even where that difference may not be destined to occur. In an effort, to avoid even the *possibility* of disorders, some parents may wish to abort or let die those children whose genomic characterizations are ambiguous. The moral question worth taking away from considerations of this kind is this: will the genomic project cast a hermeneutic of suspicion over all people and especially children? How many tests will a man have to pass to be judged fit for employment and the resultant social and personal benefits? How many tests will a woman have to pass to buy health or life insurance? How many tests will a child have to pass to be wanted, born, and loved?

One other aspect of the question worth considering here is whether or not the genome project will offer a way to conform people to the existing social order. This longstanding concern about the "engineering" of people is surely relevant to the genome project if people themselves are viewed as burdens when it is the design of society's institutions that is at fault in meeting social needs, in meeting the needs of people as they actually exist with all their diseases, defects, and differences. The question is whether the genome project will be put to the use of establishing genetic difference as personal fallibility rather than as a shared aspect of human finitude.

Regardless of the use of genomic characterizations and reproductive interventions, what of persons with genetic liabilities who are born nevertheless? Will they be seen as failures of the system, as an incentive to expand the use of genetic profiling prenatally or at birth? Or as an incentive to routine, even compulsory, genomic profiling? Will they be seen as indictments of the nation's health policy? Will they be further stigmatized as drains on society and failures in themselves because their birth defects were in principle avoidable? And how, in such circumstances, can the presumption of social equality be preserved?

It is not only in these ways that people's lives and differences are stake here. The question of the moral responsibilities of parents is also implicated insofar as the existence of genetic characterizations might also raise the threshold of responsible parenthood. How, for example, should parents who decline or resist such testing for eliminable or treatable genetic disease be seen? Will they be seen as exercising rights properly their own or as misguided people punishing their own children to advance their own private beliefs? Will their actions invite legislatures and courts to impose standards of care here? It is also worth wondering whether the availability of genomic characterizations will widen the gap between have and have-not parents. Will genetic disease become another affliction of the poor?

All these issues implicate the question of how we will understand and interpret difference. The self is bordered by differences that are essential to individuation; marking difference is an irreducible component of individuation. And it is the meaning of difference that I regard as a central moral question of the human genome project. The question is whether we will find in genetic characterizations differences that divide us further even as we lift the burden of genetic suffering. To be sure, I do not wish anyone to suffer from genetic disease for the mere sake of maintaining difference; but I do hope that we can preserve the lessons of those differences as lessons otherwise unlearned.

CONCLUSIONS

In 1660, French philosopher and mathematician Blaise Pascal wrote an essay called "Prayer to Ask God for the Right Use of Sickness."[13] The title here is problematic to contemporary consciousness. The right use of sickness? What could this signify? That if there is a right use of sickness, there is also a wrong use of sickness? That there is a purpose to sickness at all? However strange the questions might appear today, in Pascal's view, sickness could be put to the use of personal transformation and was useful in guiding one to correct moral priorities.

It is fair to say, in contrast, that the operational interpretation of contemporary biomedicine, reflecting our own pervasive social judgment, is that disease and suffering are evils to be resisted, threats to our happiness, events without meaning that we would do better to extinguish and avoid because there is nothing to learn from then, no purpose, no achievement in their endurance. But whatever else they may or may not be, suffering and other marks of difference teach us lessons not otherwise available about the nature and meaning of our lives. There is, of course, absurd suffering and pointless difference. But it is also true that we do not know what our lives are worth if we do not countenance the price we would be willing to pay for them, the difference we would be willing to endure for them.

The question before us then is one Pascal would have understood: what is the right use of the human genome project? Will it be used to prop the existing scientific status quo and perhaps thereby impede the aims of science? Will it be used in a campaign against difference, or will it be used to map the fullness and plenitude of existence? Will it be used as a stratagem to create a new kind of inferiority? Or will we be able to understand the way in which genomic characterizations represent one possible map of a small corner of the vastness of existence? Will the goal of biomedicine be the leveling of all genetic difference in order to accommodate the social requirements of the time?

It seems to me that we should not lose sight of some of the fundamental paradoxes of science as we consider judgment on the genome project. Even as it offers some answers, science also creates uncertainty; even as it conquers some social evils, it also may cause evasion of social problems. While science opens vistas of the world to our experience, it also imposes standards of conformity in scientists and what they study. And it not only offers an explanation but also advances a cause.

As a matter of moral analysis, it seems important to make the case that the differences identified by genomic mapping should not be used as a pretext for vilification, whether that vilification is couched in the language of racial impurity or human health; that the social needs of the day not be mistaken as ultimate human needs; and that we do not demand answers from the genome project to questions for which it has no authority. I hope instead that we continue to recognize that differences among individuals are rare and important goods, that the genetically atypical are important scientific and moral resources, that there is in individual human and social life a plenitude of difference that should be preserved, and that there are lessons in difference and suffering it would be unwise to bypass altogether.

In the *Pensées*, Pascal remarked that "knowledge of physical science will not console me for ignorance of morality in time of affliction, but knowledge of morality will always console me for ignorance of physical science."[14] I take Pascal to have meant that a knowledge of, for example, the genetic molecular processes of humans or any assemblage, however large, of simply factual information must necessarily fail in telling us what it is that we are worth, what it is that we ought to seek, and how we should live. Moral philosophy is therefore crucial because it concerns the standards by which we judge the nature and significance of our actions. The genome project will significantly enlarge the bounds of the human empire, increasing our genetic knowledge ten million fold. It will eventually offer insight into the secret motion of things. It is dubious, though, whether the genome project will enable us to effect all things possible. But given the lessons of history, it is not even clear that we should aspire to the effecting of all things possible. I think that we should not effect, even if it were possible, the extinction of difference. On the contrary, moral philosophy seems to require that we find what ways there are in the use of research projects and their consequences to preserve the lessons of difference, for it is only individual difference that can throw the moral order of the universe into relief and can let us know who in fact we are.

NOTES

1. Francis Bacon, *The New Organon* (New York: Liberal Arts Press, 1960).

2. Francis Bacon, *The Advancement of Learning and New Atlantis* (London: Oxford, 1974).

3. Ibid., 228.

4. Alexander M. Capron, "Which Ills to Bear? Reevaluating the 'Threat' of Modern Genetics," *Emory Law Journal* 39 (1990): 679.

5. See Loane Skene, "Mapping the Human Genome: Some Thoughts for Those Who Say There Ought To Be a Law on It," *Bioethics* 5 (1991): 233–249.

6. James D. Watson and Robert Mullan Cook-Deegan, "The Human Genome Project and International Health," *Journal of the American Medical Association* 263 (1990): 3322–3324.

7. Paul Feyerabend, *Against Method, Outline of an Anarchist Theory of Knowledge* (London: Verso, 1975).

8. Ibid.

9. Leon R. Kass, *Toward a More Natural Science* (New York: Free Press, 1985), 176.

10. Friedrich Nietzsche, *Daybreak, Thoughts on the Prejudices of Morality*, R. J. Hollingdale, trans. (Cambridge: Cambridge University Press, 1982), 134.

11. See Daniel J. Kevles, *In the Name of Eugenics: Genetics and the Uses of Human Heredity* (New York: Knopf, 1985).

12. Margaret Sanger, *The Pivot of Civilization* (Elmsford, NY: Maxwell Reprint, 1969 [originally published, 1922]).

13. Blaise Pascal, "Prière de Blaise Pascal pour demander à Dieu le bon Usage des Maladies," *Oeuvres*, Vol. IX (Paris: Librairie Hachette, 1914), 319–340.

14. Blaise Pascal, *Pensées*, A. J. Krailsheimer, trans. (London: Penguin, 1966), 36.

2

EUGENICS AND THE HUMAN GENOME PROJECT
Is the Past Prologue?

Daniel J. Kevles

In April 1991, an exposition opened in the hall atop the great arch of *La Défense* in Paris under the title *La Vie en Kit* [Life in a Test Tube]: *Éthique et Biologie*. The biological exhibits included displays about molecular genetics and the human genome project. The ethical worries were manifest in a catalog statement by the writer Monette Vaquin that was also prominently placarded at the genome display:

> Today, astounding paradox, the generation following Nazism is giving the world the tools of eugenics beyond the wildest Hitlerian dreams. It is as if the unthinkable of the generation of the fathers haunted the discoveries of the sons. Scientists of tomorrow will have a power that exceeds all the powers known to mankind: that of manipulating the genome. Who can say for sure that it will be used only for the avoidance of hereditary illnesses?[1]

Vaquin's apprehensions, echoed frequently by scientists and social analysts alike, indicate that the shadow of eugenics hangs over any discussion of the social implications of human genetics, but particularly over consideration of the potential impact of the human genome project. People wonder whether the eugenic past forms a prologue to the human genetic future.

HISTORY OF EUGENICS

Eugenic ideas go back at least to Plato, but in its modern version, eugenics originated with Francis Galton, a younger first cousin of

14

Charles Darwin and a brilliant scientist in his own right. In the late nineteenth century, Galton proposed that the human race might be improved in the manner of plant and animal breeding—that is, by getting rid of so-called undesirables and multiplying the so-called desirables. It was Galton who named this program of human improvement *eugenics:* he took the word from a Greek root meaning "good in birth" or "noble in heredity." Galton intended eugenics to improve human stock by giving "the more suitable races or strains of blood a better chance of prevailing speedily over the less suitable."[2]

Galton's eugenic ideas took popular hold after the turn of this century, developing a large following in the United States, Britain, Germany, and many other countries. Eugenic organizations were formed, including, in 1923, the American Eugenics Society, which, among other things, annually mounted eugenic exhibits at state fairs. The backbone of the movement was formed of people drawn from the white middle and upper middle classes, especially prominent laymen and scientists, particularly geneticists and often physicians. Eugenicists declared themselves to be concerned with preventing social degeneration, whose abundant signs they found in the social and behavioral discordances of urban industrial society. For example, they took crime, slums, and rampant disease to be symptoms of social pathologies, and they attributed them primarily to biological causes—that is, to "blood," to use the term of inheritable essence popular at the turn of the century.[3]

To eugenically minded biologists, the causes of social degeneration were understood as matters to be rooted out, which led some of them to pursue research in human heredity related to eugenics. As a result, the human genetics research program of the day included the study of medical disorders, such as diabetes and epilepsy, not only for their intrinsic interest but also because of their social costs. A still more substantial part of the program consisted of the analysis of traits alleged to create social burdens—traits involving qualities of temperament and behavior that might lie at the bottom of, for example, alcoholism, prostitution, criminality, and poverty. A major object of scrutiny was mental deficiency, then commonly termed "feeblemindedness," which was often identified by intelligence tests and was widely interpreted to be at the root of many varieties of socially deleterious behavior.

In the hope of explaining these pathologies biologically, eugenic researchers resorted to Mendel's laws of heredity, which had been rediscovered in 1900, fastening on the idea that biological characteristics were determined by single elements (which were later identified with genes). Their research was pervaded by the fundamental assumption that not only could such physical characteristics as eye color and disease be explained in a Mendelian fashion but so also could characteristics of mind and behavior. The assumption was embraced by Charles B. Davenport, a prominent American biologist, eugenicist, and head of the biological laboratory that, in 1918, became the Carnegie Institution of Washington's Department of Genetics at Cold Spring Harbor on Long Island, New York. Davenport searched for Mendelian patterns of inheritance in many behavioral categories, including the inheritance of what he called "nomadism," "shiftlessness," and "thalassophilia"—the love of the sea that he discerned in naval officers and concluded must be a sex-linked recessive trait because, like color blindness, it was almost always expressed in males. A chart displayed at the Kansas Free Fair in 1929, purporting to illustrate the "laws" of Mendelian inheritance in human beings, declared, "Unfit human traits such as feeblemindedness, epilespy, criminality, insanity, alcoholism, pauperism, and many others run in families and are inherited in exactly the same way as color in guinea pigs."[4]

Some eugenic investigation into human heredity proved to be meritorious, revealing, for example, that Huntington's chorea results from a dominant gene and albinism from a recessive one. However, much of it was recognized in the end to be worthless. Combining Mendelian theory with incautious speculation, eugenic scientists often neglected polygenic complexities in favor of single-gene explanations. They also paid far too little attention to cultural, economic, and other environmental influences in their accounts of mental abilities such as low scores on IQ tests and social behaviors such as prostitution. Like Davenport's behavorial categories, many of the traits that figured in eugenic research were vague or ludicrous.

Class and race prejudice were pervasive in eugenic science. In northern Europe and the United States, eugenics expressed standards of fitness and social value that were predominantly white, middle class, Protestant, and identified with "Aryans." In the reasoning of eugenicists, lower income groups were not poor because they had inadequate educational and economic opportunity but because their moral and educational capacities, rooted in their biology, were inadequate. When eugenicists celebrated Aryans, they demonstrated nothing more than their own racial biases. Davenport, indulging in unsupportable anthropology, found the Poles to be "independent and self-reliant though clannish"; the Italians tending to "crimes of personal violence"; and the Hebrews "intermediate between the slovenly Servians and the Greeks and the tidy Swedes, German, and Bohemians" and giving to "thieving" though rarely to "personal violence." He expected that the "great influx of blood from Southeastern Europe" would rapidly make the American population "darker in pigmentation, smaller in stature, more mercurial . . . more given to crimes of larceny, kidnapping, assault, murder, rape, and sex-immorality."[5]

Eugenicists such as Davenport urged interference in human propagation so as to increase the frequency of socially "good" genes in the population and decrease that of "bad" ones. The interference was to take two forms: one was "positive" eugenics, which meant manipulating human heredity and/or breeding to produce superior people, and the other was "negative" eugenics, which meant improving the quality of the human race by eliminating biologically inferior people from the population. The elimination might be accomplished by discouraging biologically inferior human beings from reproducing or entering one's own population.

In practice, little was done for positive eugenics, although eugenic claims did figure in the advent of family allowance policies in Britain and Germany during the 1930s, and positive eugenic themes were certainly implied in the so-called Fitter Family competitions that were a standard feature of eugenic programs at 1920s state fairs. These competitions were held at the fairs in the "human stock" section. At the 1924 Kansas Free Fair, for example, winning families in the three categories—small, average, and large—were awarded a Governor's Fitter Family Trophy, which was presented by Governor Jonathan Davis, and "Grade A Individuals" received a medal that portrayed two diaphanously garbed parents, their arms outstretched toward their (presumably) eugenically meritorious infant. It is hard to know what made these families and individuals stand out as fit, but some evidence is supplied by the fact that all entrants had to take an IQ test—and the Wasserman test for syphilis.[6]

Much more was done for negative eugenics, notably the passage of eugenic sterilization laws. By the late 1920s, some two dozen American states had enacted such laws. The laws were declared constitutional in the 1927 U.S. Supreme Court decision of *Buck v. Bell*, in which Justice Oliver Wendell Holmes delivered the opinion that three generations of imbeciles were enough. The leading state in this endeavor was California, which as of 1933 had subjected more people to eugenic sterilization than had all other states of the union combined.[7]

The most powerful union of eugenic research and public policy occurred in Nazi Germany. Much of eugenic research in Germany before and even during the Nazi period was similar to that in the United States and Britain, but during the Hitler years, Nazi bureaucrats provided eugenic research institutions with handsome support. Their research programs were expanded to complement the goals of Nazi biological policy, exploiting ongoing investigations into the inheritance of disease, intelligence, and behavior to advise the government on its sterilization policy. A major eugenics institute, the staff of which included the prominent geneticist Otmar von Verschuer, trained doctors for the SS in the intricacies of racial hygiene and analyzed data and specimens obtained in the concentration camps. Some of the material—for example, the internal organs of dead children and the skeletons of two murdered Jews—came from Josef Mengele, who had been a graduate student of Verschuer's and was his assistant at the institute. In 1942, Verschuer became head of the institute (he would go on to serve postwar Germany as professor of human genetics at the University of Muenster).[8] In Germany, where sterilization measures were partly inspired by the California law, the eugenics movement prompted the sterilization of several hundred thousand people and helped lead to the death camps.

EUGENIC PROSPECTS

Since the opening of the DNA era, observers have wondered whether new genetic knowledge will be deployed for positive eugenics, for attempts to produce a super race or at least to engineer new Einsteins, Mozarts, or athletes such as Kareem Abdul-Jabbar. (Curiously, brilliantly talented women, such as Marie Curie, Nadia Boulanger, or athletes such as Martina Navratilova, are rarely if ever mentioned in the pantheon of superpeople.) Conferences on the human genome project almost inevitably produce expressions of fear that the state will seek to foster or enhance a variety of highly valued human qualities or characteristics.

The apprehensions are not entirely unfounded given certain recent events. In Singapore in 1984, for example, Prime Minister Lee Kwan Yew deplored the relatively low birth rate among educated women, contending that their intelligence was higher than average and that they were thus allowing the quality of the country's gene pool to diminish. Since then, that government, embracing a crude positive eugenics, has adopted a variety of incentives, such as preferential school enrollment for offspring, to increase fecundity among such women and has provided similar incentives to their less educated sisters who will have themselves sterilized after the birth of a first or second child.[9]

However, it is doubtful that advances in genetic knowledge will lead to a revival of attempts to produce a super race. While the human genome project will undoubtedly accelerate the identification of genes for physical and medical traits, it is unlikely to reveal with any speed how genes contribute to the formation of those qualities— talent, behavior, personality—that the world admires. Equally important, the engineering of designer human genomes is not possible under current reproductive technologies and is not likely to grow much easier in the near future.

Many more commentators, such as the late Nobel laureate biologist Salvador Luria, and advocates of rights for the disabled, such as Barbara Faye Waxman, have cautioned that the human genome project is likely to foster a revival of negative eugenics. Since it will in principle be easy to identify individuals with deleterious genes of a physical (or presumptively antisocial) type, the state may intervene in reproductive behavior so as to discourage the transmission of these genes in the population. Indeed, in 1988, China's Gansu Province adopted a eugenic law that would (so the authorities said) improve "population quality" by banning the marriages of mentally retarded people unless they first submit to sterilization. Since then, such laws have been adopted in other provinces and have been endorsed by Prime Minister Li Peng. The official newspaper *Peasants Daily* explained, "Idiots give birth to idiots."[10]

Negative eugenics appeared to motivate the European Commission when, in July 1988, it proposed the creation of a human genome project for the European Community.[11] Called a health measure, the proposal was entitled "Predictive Medicine: Human Genome Analysis." Its rationale rested on a simple syllogism—that many diseases result from interactions of genes and environment; that it would be impossible to remove all the environmental culprits from society; and that, hence, individuals could be better defended against disease by identifying their genetic predispositions to fall ill. According to the summary of the proposal, "Predictive Medicine seeks to protect individuals from the kinds of illnesses to which they are genetically most vulnerable and, where appropriate, to prevent the transmission of the genetic susceptibilities to the next generation."[12]

In the view of the Commission, the genome proposal, which it found to be consistent with the European Community's main objectives for research and development, would enhance the quality of life by decreasing the prevalence of many diseases distressful to families and expensive to European society. In the long term, it would make Europe more competitive—indirectly by helping to slow the rate of increase in health expenditures, and directly by strengthening its scientific and technological base. To the end of fostering European prosperity by creating a "Europe of health," the Commission proposed to establish a modest Community human genome project, providing it with 15 million ECU (about $17 million) for the three years beginning January 1, 1989.[13]

Economics may well prove to be a powerful incentive to a new negative eugenics. Undoubtedly, concern for financial costs played a role in the eugenics movement. The social pathologies of the early twentieth century were said to be increasing at a costly rate. At the Sesquicentennial Exposition in Philadelphia in 1926, for example, the American Eugenics Society exhibit included a board that, in the manner of the population counters of a later day, revealed with flashing lights that every fifteen seconds a hundred dollars of your money went for the care of people with bad heredity, that every forty-eight seconds a mentally deficient person was born in the United States, and that only every seven and a half minutes did the United States enjoy the birth of "a high-grade person . . . who will have ability to do creative work and be fit for leadership." Thus, it was reasoned, eliminate bad genes from the gene pool and you would reduce what are now called state and local welfare costs, by reducing public expenditures for "feeblemindedness" in its public institutional settings—that is, state institutions and state hospitals for the mentally deficient and physically disabled or diseased. Perhaps indicative of this reasoning is that, in California and several other states, eugenic sterilization rates increased significantly during the 1930s when state budgets for the mentally handicapped were squeezed.[14]

In our own day, the more that health care in the United States becomes a public responsibility, payable through the tax system, and the more expensive this care becomes, the greater the possibility that taxpayers will rebel against paying for the care of those whom genetics dooms to severe disease or disability. To be sure, the more that is learned about the human genome, the more it will become obvious that we are all susceptible to certain kinds of genetic diseases or disabilities, that we all carry some genetic load and are likely to fall sick in one way or another. Since everyone is in jeopardy of genetically based illness, then everyone would have an interest in a well-financed public health program—national health insurance—and everyone would have a stake in extending its benefits universally. However, not everyone's genetic load is the same; some are more severe and costly than others. It is likely that, on grounds of cost, even a national health system might seek to discriminate among patients, using the criterion of how expensive their therapy and care might be. Public policy might feel pressure to encourage, or even compel, people not to bring genetically affected children into the world—not for the sake of the gene pool but in the interest of keeping public health costs down.

All this said, however, a number of factors are likely to offset a scenario of socially controlled reproduction, let alone a revival of broad-based negative eugenics. Analysts of civil liberty know that reproductive freedom is much more easily curtailed in dictatorial governments than in democratic ones. Eugenics profits from authoritarianism—indeed, almost requires it. The institutions of political democracy may not have been robust enough to resist altogether the violations of civil liberties characteristic of the early eugenics movement, but they did contest them effectively in many places. The British government refused to pass eugenic sterilization laws. So did many American states, and where they were enacted, they were often unenforced. It is far-fetched to expect a Nazi-like eugenics program to develop in the contemporary United States as long as political democracy and the Bill of Rights continue in force. If a Nazi-like eugenics program becomes a threatening reality, the country will have a good deal more to worry about politically than just eugenics.

What makes contemporary political democracies unlikely to embrace eugenics is that they contain powerful antieugenic constituencies. Awareness of the barbarities and cruelties of state-sponsored eugenics in the past has tended to set most geneticists and the public at large against such programs. Most geneticists today know better than their early twentieth century predecessors that ideas concerning what is "good for the gene pool" are highly problematic. Also, handicapped and diseased persons are politically empowered, as are minority groups, to a degree that they were not in the early twentieth century. They may not be sufficiently empowered to counter all quasi-eugenic threats to themselves, but they are politically positioned, with allies in the media, the medical profession, and the Roman Catholic Church—a staunch opponent of the eugenics movement—to block or at least to hinder eugenics proposals that might affect them.[15]

An antieugenic coalition rose up in response to the European Commission's proposal for a human genome project for predictive medicine after it went to the European Parliament for consideration. In the Parliament, primary responsibility for evaluating the genome proposal was given on September 12, 1988, to the Committee on Energy, Research and Technology, which considered it in several meetings and, by late January 1989, was ready to vote on a report concerning the matter.[16] The drafting of committee reports in the Parliament is guided by a member, a rapporteur, who is designated for the purpose and who can exercise enormous influence over the position that the committee eventually adopts. The rapporteur appointed for the genome proposal was Benedikt Härlin, a Green Party member from what was then West Germany. Opposition to genetic engineering has been widespread there, and it has been especially sharp among the Greens, a disparate coalition united mainly by a common interest in environmental protection. The Greens' desire to preserve nature has been suffused with distrust of technology and suspicion of human genetic manipulations. The Greens had helped impose severe restrictions on biotechnology in West Germany and raised objections to human genome research on grounds that it might lead to a recrudescence of Nazi biological policies. As James Burn, a Scottish expert on biotechnology and a longtime resident of West Germany, once told a reporter, "Germans have an abiding and understandable fear of anything to do with genetic research. It is the one science that reminds them all of everything they want to forget."[17]

The Härlin report, insisting that the European Community remember, raised a red flag against the genome project as an enterprise in preventive medicine. It reminded the Community that, in the past, eugenic ideas had led to "horrific consequences" and declared that "clear pointers to eugenic tendencies and goals" were inherent in the intention of protecting people from contracting and transmitting genetic diseases. The application of human genetic information for such purposes would almost always involve decisions, fundamentally eugenic ones, about what are "normal and abnormal, acceptable and unacceptable, viable and non-viable forms of the genetic make-up of individual human beings before and after birth." The Härlin report also warned that the new biological and reproductive technologies could make for a "modern test tube eugenics," a eugenics all the more insidious because it could disguise more easily than its cruder ancestors "an even more radical and totalitarian form of 'biopolitics'." Holding that the primary function of a European health and research policy must be "to block any eugenic trends in relation to human genome research," the report judged the proposed program in predictive medicine "unacceptable" as it stood.[18]

Härlin actually wished to make it acceptable, not to reject it. ("You can't keep Germany out of the future," he later said about his own country's involvement in genome research.[19]) On January 25, 1989, the energy committee voted twenty to one to adopt the Härlin report. It thus urged Parliament's endorsement of the European Commission's proposal as it would be modified by thirty-eight amendments contained in the report, including the complete excision of the phrase "predictive medicine" from the text. Collectively, the modifications were mainly designed to exclude a eugenically oriented health policy; to prohibit research seeking to modify the human germ line; to protect the privacy and anonymity of individual genetic data; and to ensure ongoing debate into the social, ethical, and legal dimensions of human genetic research.[20]

In mid-February 1989, the Härlin report whisked through a first reading in the European Parliament, drawing support not only from the Greens but also from conservatives on both sides of the English Channel, including German Catholics. The Parliament's action prompted Filip Maria Pandolfi, the new European Commissioner for Research and Development, in early April 1989 to freeze indefinitely Community human genome monies. The move was believed to be the first by a commissioner to block one of Brussels' own technological initiatives. Pandolfi explained that time for reflection was needed because "when you have British conservatives agreeing with German Greens, you know it's a matter of concern."[21]

The reflection produced, in mid-November, a modified proposal from the European Commission that accepted the thrust of the amendments and even the language of a number of them. The new proposal called for a three-year program of human genome analysis as such, without regard to predictive medicine, and committed the Community in a variety of ways—most notably, by prohibiting human germ line research and genetic intervention with human embryos—to avoid eugenic practices, prevent ethical missteps, and protect individual rights and privacy. It also promised to keep the Parliament and the public fully informed via annual reports on the moral and legal basis of human genome research.[22] On December 15, 1989, the modified proposal was adopted by the European Community Council of Ministers as its common position on the genome project. The Parliament having raised no objections, on June 29, 1990, the common position was promulgated by the Council as the human genome program of the Community, authorized for three years at a total cost of 15 million ECU, seven percent of which was designated for ethical studies.[23]

THE REAL SOCIAL CHALLENGES

The eugenic past is prologue to the human genetic future in only a strictly temporal sense, that is, it came before. Of course, the imagined prospects and possibilities of human genetic engineering remain tantalizing, even if they are still largely the stuff of science fiction, and they will continue to elicit both fearful condemnation and enthusiastic speculation. However, the near-term ethical challenges of the human genome project lie neither in private forays in human genetic improvement nor in some state-mandated program of eugenics. They lie in the grit of what the project will produce in abundance: genetic information. They center on the control, diffusion, and use of that information within the context of a market economy, and they are deeply troubling.

The advance of human genetics and biotechnology has created the capacity for a kind of "homemade eugenics," to use the insightful term of the analyst Robert Wright—"individual families deciding what kinds of kids they want to have." At the moment, the kinds they can select are those without certain disabilities or diseases, such as Down's syndrome or Tay–Sachs. Most parents would probably prefer just a healthy baby, if they are inclined to choose at all. But in the future, some might have the opportunity, via genetic analysis of embryos, to have improved babies, children who are likely to be more intelligent or more athletic or better looking (whatever those comparative terms mean).

Will people pursue such opportunities? Quite possibly, given the interest that some parents have shown in choosing the sex of their child or in administering growth hormone to offspring who they think will grow up too short. Benedikt Härlin's report to the European Parliament on the human genome project noted that the increasing availability of genetic tests was generating increasingly widespread pressure from families for "individual eugenic choice in order to give one's own child the best possible start in a society in which heredity traits become a criterion of social hierarchy." A 1989 editorial in *Trends in Biotechnology* recognized a major source of the pressure: " 'Human improvement' is a fact of life, not because of the state eugenics committee, but because of consumer demand. How can we expect to deal responsibly with human genetic information in such a culture?"[24]

The increasing availability of human genetic information challenges individuals with wrenching decisions. Purely for personal reasons, people may not wish to obtain their genetic profiles, particularly if they are at risk for an inheritable disease for which no treatment is known. Still, genetic testing, prenatal or otherwise, can be liberating if it reveals to individuals that either they or their newly conceived children are free from some specific genetic doom. A young woman tested and found to lack the gene for Huntington's declared, "After 28 years of not knowing, it's like being released from prison. To have hope for the future . . . to be able to see my grandchildren."[25]

The problems and opportunities of individual choices aside, the torrent of new human genetic information will undoubtedly pose

challenges to systems and values of social decency. Much of the discussion on this point has rightly emphasized that employers may seek
to deny jobs to applicants with a susceptibility (or alleged susceptibility) to disorders such as manic depression or illnesses arising from
features of the workplace. Life and medical insurance companies may
well wish to know the genomic signatures of their clients, their profile
of risk for disease and death. Even national health systems might
choose to ration the provision of care on the basis of genetic pro-
pensity for disease, especially to families at risk for bearing diseased
children.

Many analysts have contended that individual genomic information should be protected as strictly private. However, a great deal
more thought needs to be given to the rights of individuals to withhold and the rights of insurers to demand such information. Insurance and insurance premiums depend on assessments of risk. If degree of risk can be concealed, it is not insurance companies as such
that will bear the costs, but other policy holders. In short, it could be
that classes of people with low risk will be compelled to subsidize
classes of others at higher risk. Thus, insisting on a right to privacy
in genetic information could well lead—at least under the system of
insurance that now prevails in the United States—to inequitable consequences.

The eugenic past has much to teach about how to avoid repeating
its mistakes, not to mention its sins. But what bedeviled our forebears
will not necessarily vex us, certainly not in the same ways. In human
genetics, as in so many others areas of life, the flow of history compels
us to think and act anew. It is important not to become absorbed
with exaggerated fears that the human genome project will foster a
drive for the production of superbabies or the callous elimination of
the unfit. It is essential to focus on the genuine social, ethical, and
policy issues—some of them already evident—that the human genome project raises, and to respond to them by creating codes of law
and/or regulation for the use of human genetic information by geneticists, the media, insurers, employers, and the government itself.

NOTES

1. *La Vie en Kit: Éthique et Biologie* (Paris: L'Arche de la Défense, 1991),
25. "Aujourd'hui, stupéfiant paradoxe, la génération qui suit le nazisme

donne au monde les outils de l'eugénisme au-delà des rêves hitlériens les plus fous. Comme si l'impensé de la génération des pères hantait les découvertes des fils. Les scientifiques de demain auront un pouvoir qui excède tous les pouvoirs connus dans l'humanité: celui de manipuler le génome. Qui peut jurer qu'il ne servira qu'à l'évitement des maladies héréditaires?"

2. Francis Galton, *Inquiries into the Human Faculty* (London: Macmillan, 1883), 24–25; Karl Pearson, *The Life, Letters, and Labours of Francis Galton* (3 vols. in 4; Cambridge, U.K.: Cambridge University Press, 1914–1930), IIIA, 348.

3. Historical accounts of eugenics, which itself produced a vast literature, have multiplied in recent years. For treatments of the subject in the United States and Britain, see Daniel J. Kevles, *In the Name of Eugenics: Genetics and the Uses of Human Heredity* (New York: Alfred A. Knopf, 1985) and G. R. Searle, *Eugenics and Politics in Britain, 1900–1914* (Leyden: Noordhoff International Publishing, 1976). For Germany, see Benno Müller-Hill, *Murderous Science: Elimination by Scientific Selection of Jews, Gypsies, and Others, Germany, 1933–1945* (New York: Oxford University Press, 1988); Robert N. Proctor, *Racial Hygiene: Medicine Under the Nazis* (Cambridge, MA: Harvard University Press, 1988); Sheila Faith Weiss, *Race Hygiene and National Efficiency: The Eugenics of Wilhelm Schallmayer* (Berkeley: University of California Press, 1987); and Paul Weindling, *Health, Race and German Politics between National Unification and Nazism, 1870–1945* (Cambridge, U.K.: Cambridge University Press, 1990).

4. Kevles, *In the Name of Eugenics*, 62; Kenneth M. Ludmerer, *Genetics and American Society: A Historical Appraisal* (Baltimore, MD: Johns Hopkins University Press, 1972), 60.

5. Charles B. Davenport, *Heredity in Relation to Eugenics* (New York: Henry Holt, 1911), 216, 218–219, 221–222.

6. Kevles, *In the Name of Eugenics*, 61–62.

7. Ibid., 107–112, 114–116; *Buck v. Bell*, 274 U.S. 201–207 (1927).

8. Proctor, *Racial Hygiene*, 44, 292, 307.

9. Stephen Jay Gould, *The Flamingo's Smile: Reflections in Natural History* (New York: W. W. Norton, 1985), 292–295, 301–303.

10. *New York Times*, 15 August 1991, p. 1.

11. The Commission is the Brussels-based executive arm of the European Community (the term has come to replace the phrase *European Communities*, meaning the European Economic Community, the European Coal and Steel Community, and the European Atomic Energy Community). It described its proposal as "a European response to the international challenges presented by the large-scale biological research projects in the United States . . . and Japan (Human Frontier Science Programme)," adding, "Although it is a programme of basic precompetitive research, both new information and

new materials of potential commercial value will result; new technological processes will also be developed. These will all contribute to the development of Europe's biotechnology industry—often based in small and medium-sized enterprises." Commission of the European Communities, *Proposal for a Council Decision Adopting a Specific Research Programme in the Field of Health; Predictive Medicine: Human Genome Analysis (1989–1991)*, COM (88) 424 final-SYN 146, Brussels, 20 July 1988, 1.

12. Ibid., 3.

13. Ibid., 10, 12, 20, 30.

14. Kevles, *In the Name of Eugenics,* 62–63; Philip R. Reilly, *The Surgical Solution: A History of Involuntary Sterilization in the United States* (Baltimore: The Johns Hopkins University Press, 1991), 91–93. The last state eugenic sterilization law was passed in 1937, in Georgia, partly in response to conditions of overcrowding in the state's institutions for the mentally handicapped. Edward J. Larson, "Breeding Better Georgians," *Georgia Journal of Southern Legal History* 1 (1991): 53–79.

15. The Roman Catholic Church took an official stand against eugenics in 1930, in the Papal Encyclical *Casti Connubii* (Kevles, *In the Name of Eugenics,* 119). The Church's well-known opposition to abortion sets it against the kind of eugenics that spokespeople for the handicapped currently fear since such a eugenics can be accomplished at the moment only by the abortion of fetuses determined to be "defective" by amniocentesis, ultrasound, or some combination of the two.

16. European Parliament, Committee on Energy, Research, and Technology, *Report Drawn up on Behalf of the Committee on Energy, Research and Technology on the Proposal from the Commission to the Council (COM/88/424-C2-119/ 88) for a Decision Adopting a Specific Research Programme in the Field of Health; Predictive Medicine: Human Genome Analysis (1989–1991)*. Rapporteur Benedikt Härlin, European Parliament Session Documents, 1988–89, 30.01.1989, Series A, Doc. A2-0370/88 SYN 146, p.3. Auxiliary opinions were also requested of the Committee on Budgets and the Committee on the Environment, Public Health, and Consumer Protection.

17. *Financial Times* [London], 10 May 1989, p. 18; Joel Davis, *Mapping the Code: The Human Genome Project and the Choices of Modern Science* (New York: John Wiley & Sons, 1990), 175; Michael Specter, "Petunias Survive German Debate over Biotechnology," *International Herald Tribune,* 12 April 1990. The German fear of genetics and eugenics would intensify, leading some activist groups on a number of occasions to intimidate and even suppress debate on biomedical subjects in universities using methods reminiscent of the Nazis (Peter Singer, "On Being Silenced in Germany," *The New York Review of Books,* 15 August 1991, pp. 36–42).

18. European Parliament, *Report on Proposal,* 23–28.

19. Specter, "German Debate over Biotechnology."

20. European Parliament, *Report on Proposal*, 3, 5–7,10–11,14. Härlin's committee was strongly supported in its position by the Committee on the Environment, Public Health, and Consumer Protection, which recommended modification of the genome project proposal to the end that the medical, ethical, legal, and social implications of such research be investigated before any specific technical projects were promoted or continued. To the Committee's members, it was "quite clear that ethical problems will arise, particularly concerning eugenic problems and access to information by individuals, States, employers, insurance companies (etc.), if the programme is successful in its long term ambitions." (Committee on the Environment, Public Health, and Consumer Protection, *Opinion for the Committee on Energy, Research, and Technology on the Proposal from the Commission of the European Communities for a Council Decision Adopting a Specific Research Programme in the Field of Health; Predictive Medicine: Human Genome Analysis (1989–1991)*, (COM/88/424 final-SYN 146-Doc. C2-119/88), 3, 5–8).

21. *Financial Times* [London], 5 April 1989, BioDoc: A collection of documents on biotechnology, European Economic Community, DG-XII, Brussels; Dirk Stemerding, "Political Decision-Making on Human Genome Research in Europe," paper delivered at Harvard workshop on the Human Genome Project, 15 June 1990, 2.

22. Commission of the European Communities, *Modified Proposal for a Council Decision, Adopting a Specific Research and Technological Development Programme in the Field of Health: Human Genome Analysis, (1990–1991)*, 13 November 1989, pp. 2–4, 11–17; *Scrip*, 8 December 1989, p. 5; copy in BioDoc.

23. European Community, *Common Position Adopted by the Council on 15 December 1989, . . . Programme in the Field of Health: Human Genome Analysis (1990–1991)*, Brussels, 15 Dec. 1989, 10619/89; *Official Journal of the European Communities*, No. L 196/8, 26/7/90, Council Decision of 29 June 1990, adopting a specific research and technological development programme in the field of health, human genome analysis (1990–1991), (90/395/EEC).

24. Jane E. Brody, "Personal Health," *New York Times*, 8 November 1990, p. B7; Barry Werth, "How Short Is Too Short?" *New York Times Magazine*, 16 June 1991, 15, 17, 28–29; European Parliament, *Report on Proposal*, 25–26; John Hodgson, "Editorial: Geneticism and Freedom of Choice," *Trends in Biotechnology*, September 1989, 221.

25. Jerry E. Bishop and Michael Waldholz, *Genome: The Story of the Most Astonishing Adventure of Our Time—The Attempt To Map All the Genes in the Human Body* (New York: Simon and Schuster, 1990), 274.

3

HANDLE WITH CARE
Race, Class, and Genetics

Arthur L. Caplan

RACE, ETHNICITY, CLASS, AND GENETICS—
A GRIM AND DISMAL HISTORY

Discussions of the consequences of increased knowledge concerning the composition and structure of the human genome for public policy often leave those involved with research or clinical care in the domain of human genetics surprised and angry. They are often taken aback by the high level of ethical concern expressed about their work. Why is it, they wonder, that knowledge of human heredity so often becomes the center of controversy and protest? Why is it that in some nations, such as Germany,[1] talk of genetic engineering or gene therapy elicits heated political protests, strict legislative controls, and sometimes outright bans on certain types of research? There can be no disputing the fact that the subject of genetics evinces a great deal of concern and worry. The reason why this is so is to be found in the past.

Human genetics has a problematic history, and sadly, minorities and the poor have not fared well in that history. Genetics, race, and ethnicity have sometimes proven to be an explosive and even fatal mixture. In Germany, for example, racial and ethnic minorities paid with their lives when developments in genetics were used in the service of a science of racial hygiene whose leaders gave enthusiastic and vocal support to Nazism.[2] Groups such as Jews, Gypsies, and Slavs were targeted for extermination on the grounds that their genes posed a threat to the overall health and reproductive well-being of the German people.

Some dismiss Nazi science as merely mad science or bad science,[3]

30

but the involvement with Nazism by many mainstream authorities and leaders in medicine, public health, and science in a technologically and scientifically advanced nation cannot be dismissed as merely "fringe" or "peripheral." The road to Dachau and Auschwitz runs too straight through the eugenic institutes and genetic courts of pre–World War II Germany to be considered nothing more than an inexplicable detour.[4]

Obviously, there is no inherent connection between the science of genetics and a public policy of murder and euthanasia based upon race hygiene. Nazism or genocidal policies cannot be deduced or inferred from facts about human heredity, and it would be dangerous to suggest otherwise. But genetics, at least in the form that prevailed in Germany during the 1920s and 1930s, served as a powerful source, tool, and buttress for racist ideology—an ideology that took a terrible toll in human lives.

It is worth noting that the majority of biologists, social scientists, and physicians who used their beliefs about human heredity to support the Nazi cause were not forced to do so. Some had arrived at racist conclusions long before the Nazi party came to power.[5] They lent their support because they believed their scientific beliefs were consistent with Nazism and not because the Nazis demanded that they fit their science to suit an ideological purpose.[6] Neither biomedical science in general nor genetics in particular were responsible for the rise of the Third Reich or the Holocaust, but some scientists and physicians used their skills and authority to create a "scientific" foundation for the racism that was a pivotal factor in legitimating Nazism and bringing about the Holocaust.[7]

The case for the tie between mainstream genetics and racist social policy is bolstered by the fact that efforts to link genetics and social policy were not confined to Germany. For example, in the United States for much of the first half of this century, the mentally ill, the retarded, alcoholics, recent immigrants, and those thought to be sexually promiscuous, especially if they were members of minority groups and poor, became the object of government-sponsored sterilization efforts aimed at preventing the spread of "bad" genes to future generations.[8] Restrictive immigration laws, forced sterilization, and prohibitions on interracial marriage were in part a legacy of mixing genetics, race, and class in the United States and many other countries.

The use of genetic information to guide American social policy continued through the 1960s and 1970s with mixed results. Attempts to conduct mass screening programs to detect carriers for such diseases as sickle cell, thalassemia, and Tay–Sachs led to much confusion, misunderstanding, and stigma.[9] One state considered enacting a law requiring any child found to be a carrier of the sickle cell gene to be vaccinated before admission to public school even though this would have no possible prophylactic effect! Companies and government agencies such as the Department of Defense enacted discriminatory policies that excluded African-Americans from jobs or promotions based on flawed and confused misunderstandings about the genetic basis of disease.[10] Efforts to create mass screening programs aimed at particular groups in an atmosphere of uncertainty about the meaning of genetic information as well as prejudice and bias resulted in a great deal of harm.

Inquiry into behaviors such as criminality, intelligence, aggressiveness, homosexuality, altruism, and mathematical skill and their prevalence in various ethnic or racial groups have been and continue to be the source of heated debate within and outside the scientific community in the United States and many other nations. While careful inquiry into these subjects is certainly appropriate, it is also the case that the results of such inquiries must be handled with great caution since racism and prejudice are still with us. For example, many women continue to this day to have abortions upon learning that the fetus they are carrying is 47XYY, a condition that some geneticists maintained more than a decade ago was causally responsible for criminal conduct. While the evidence for the "criminal chromosome" has proven weak, the consequences for procreative decisions have proven to be very resilient. There are many genetics screening programs in India, Canada, and other nations that provide prenatal screening and testing services to couples seeking to abort any fetus that is female, no questions asked.[11] There is no evidence from the realm of genetics that being female is a disease. Nonetheless, genetic information can have direct and indirect consequences for female fetuses if it is simply dumped into the public arena where bias and prejudice are allowed to mix with information about heredity.

Racism, prejudice, and genetics have made for a socially combustible and often deadly mix. The mixture has proven so toxic that a strong case can be made that applying knowledge from the realm of human genetics to public policy has led to far more misery, confusion, and suffering in the twentieth century than it has to human betterment. History suggests that there are real reasons for concern about the impact a rapid increase in knowledge about human heredity might have on current and future social policy. This is especially true in light of the fact that those who proudly espouse racism continue to invoke the terminology of genetics to support their views.[12]

But is it really fair to assess the implications for human groups and populations of the human genome project solely on the basis of history? After all, Nazi racial hygiene, while accepted by many scientists of that era as valid, is understood today to be invalid. And the genetics reflected in Nazi social policy is simply an instance of biomedical information being applied in a political state gone mad. The eugenic dreams of some biologists and physicians concerning prophylactic sterilization that led to government-sponsored programs of coercive surgery in many regions of the United States combined what we now recognize as fallacious science with overt prejudice. Why should we let the errors of the past be our guide to the ethical implications of current work in genetics when we are no longer bound by crude knowledge concerning human heredity, the yoke of totalitarian ideologies or the scurrilous prejudices of our parents and grandparents?

Ironically, the only way to understand the significance of the past with respect to justice and genetics in thinking about the implications of the human genome project for various groups and subpopulations may be to look forward into the future. By trying to imagine how our own (hypothetically) more sophisticated (at least hypothetically), more humane (at least arguably), and tolerant values (at least hypothetically) might combine with new, less error-laden (at least hypothetically) genetic knowledge to produce a range of consequences for various groups thirty or fifty years from now, we might be in a better position to evaluate the lessons taught by historical experiences of the past.

FUTURE IMPLICATIONS OF THE GENOME PROJECT FOR MINORITIES AND GROUPS

Imagine that the year is 2030. It is ten years after the completion of the complete genome maps for human beings, fruit flies, slime molds, carp, the roundworm, the Norway rat, the dog, the chimpanzee, and a large number of viruses and bacteria. Much work has been done to try to analyze the connections between structure and function in these genomes and to examine how the information contained in the genome interacts with the environment to mediate ontogenesis across a whole range of characteristics and behaviors. Not only are a large number of *archetypal maps* on hand for a large number of animal and plant species but a large number of regional maps, called *demic maps,* have also been compiled. These provide an overview of key areas of the genome in various races and subpopulations—*demes*—in animal species and in various racial and ethnic groups in the human population. The maps provide information about the precise degree of variation that exists within subpopulations at certain key loci. The X and Y chromosomes have been analyzed down to the finest detail. What sorts of policies and issues might have evolved by this point in time? What sorts of implications would this knowledge have for equity, fairness, and justice? Consider six possible case scenarios that might be occupying the attention of bioethicists of the twenty-first century.

Case 1. Who is a Jew?

A certain Avram Kaplan has decided to immigrate from his home in Minnesota to Israel. He can no longer stand the sterile, artificially controlled climate of his home state and wants to go back to a land that has been preserved in a relatively pristine, natural, and peaceful state by international accords. He knows that, as a Jew, he has the right to return to Israel as a citizen. But he faces the problem that his grandmother on his mother's side was not Jewish.

The Orthodox rabbinate in Israel, who sets policy on matters regarding the law of return, insists that every person invoking the law of return to enter Israel as a citizen undergo genetic testing. The Israeli government maintains a large computerized registry of demic maps obtained from the genomes of Jews from various parts of the world. Whenever an immigrant arrives, a tissue sample is taken and the genetic material from the cells is used to cross-check claims of Jewish identity with the deme maps in the registry. By examining the X chromosome, it is possible to identify markers that show whether a man did or did not have a "Jewish" mother or is of Jewish matrilineal descent.

There has been much criticism of the idea within and outside of Israel that there are ideal or "typical" maps for different races or groups, but since these same maps are widely used in molecular anthropology, forensic biopsychology, and biological archeology, it is difficult to argue that the systematics used in those fields are of no utility in the realm of public policy. Many governments and the United Nations have sanctioned the use of genomic archetypes to help resolve land conflicts and ancestral ownership claims among Tibetans and Chinese, Azeris and Armenians, and Serbs and Croats, as well as those in Poland, Russia, and the Ukraine who claim German citizenship on the grounds that they are ethnic Germans. The secular law in many nations including the United States has long recognized archetypical and demic matching as legitimate techniques for establishing individual identity.

Is it fair for genetic testing to be used for the purpose of identifying who is and is not a "real" or "true" member of a racial group? Should those doing tests agree to do them for nonmedical, non-health-related reasons? Should religious authorities in nations where ancestry is seen as relevant to the religious or social standing of a person be discouraged or encouraged to use genetic testing to remove uncertainties?

Case 2. Affirmative Action

Sally Hightower was thrilled to learn that the U.S. government had started a new program to encourage Native American people to enter the field of philosophy. The demand for teachers of philosophy had escalated dramatically with the shift in demographics toward a much older society. Sally was certain she could qualify for the scholarship since she had long been active in her tribe. She was on the tribal council, had participated in numerous interviews with anthropologists and oral historians seeking to record Native American ways of life, and was one of only a handful of people remaining fluent in her tribe's language. She had long had an interest in ethics and was eager to take advantage of the opportunity to go to college.

Federal regulations required sequence matches on at least six key marker areas of one of the Native American subpopulation maps in order to qualify for the program. All applicants were required to submit a blood sample for use in determining eligibility for affirmative action programs such as this one.

When Sally's DNA was extracted from the refrigerated blood sample she sent to the Bureau of Indian Identity and Affairs, it failed to achieve the requisite number of matches. Unbeknown to her, she had quite a bit of white ancestry. The government was uncertain about what to do with respect to her application since it would be politically difficult to turn down a person as prominent in Native American affairs as Sally on the grounds that she failed to satisfy the biological test requirements federal law mandated to be classified as a Native American. Sally would also be uncertain as to what to make of these test results. Should she resign her position on the tribal council? Was she deceiving her closest friends if she chose not to reveal her white ancestry?

Is it fair to use information about the genetic makeup or composition of a population to establish membership in a racial, ethnic, or tribal group? Should social policy allow people to define themselves on the basis of culture and behavior as belonging to a particular group, or is biological inheritance a key element of membership as well? Should such tests be required for the purposes of determining eligibility for affirmative action or equal opportunity programs? Would such evidence be admitted or even required in discrimination suits?

Case 3. The Real Scoop on Jimmy Carter

By the turn of the century, so many scientists, conspiracy theory buffs, biographers, and media organizations were seeking samples of tissue of former U.S. Presidents for genetic analysis at the Smithsonian Institution that the National Presidential Tissue Sample Registry had been established with strict rules governing access, disclosure of findings, and the collection of new materials. Some samples, such as those of Lincoln and Kennedy, were of enormous interest. Others, such as those of Chester A. Arthur and Franklin Pierce, drew very little attention.

The registry had a number of thorny issues to contend with concerning the control of information about public figures. The discovery of the source of Gerald Ford's lack of balance as resulting from a congenital neurological defect had created such a stir among his descendants that the museum felt it could no longer honor every request for cells or tissues. The earlier decision by George Bush not to permit a tissue sample to be kept in the registry to protect his and his family's privacy had led the Smithsonian to call for legislation guaranteeing a fifty-year ban following the death of the source of tissues before they would be made available to the general public for analysis.

But now the museum faced a very tough problem. A researcher at Emory medical school who was interested in the genetics of the pancreatic cancer that had ultimately caused Jimmy Carter's death had inadvertently found a marker on a segment of Carter's DNA that suggested he might have had a distant relative who was African-American. Should the general public be told? How should unintentionally acquired information about race or ethnicity be handled in terms of privacy, confidentiality, and disclosure?

Case 4. Immigration and Human Disease Vectors

North American immigration authorities did not like the policy that forbids those of Haitian ancestry to enter the United States and Canada, but they enforced it. Five years earlier, it had been found using genome maps and genetic autopsies that poor Haitians of African descent were especially likely to be carriers of mitochondrial prions, which had long been implicated in the transmission of degenerative diseases such as multiple sclerosis, some forms of arthritis, some cancers, and lupus. At that time, governments all around the world restricted the rights of Haitians to visit or immigrate freely. The policy required a quick-scan genetic screen to be run on all nonwhites living outside North America to establish racial and ethnic identity and ancestry. This took time, was costly, and led to a large number of fights and arguments between immigration authorities and would-be immigrants.

The immigration authorities were not wild about having to handle and risk contact with infected or potentially infected tissue specimens. Also, it was not clear that the level of risk or danger to the public health would justify restrictions on freedom of movement for various groups and subpopulations within American society. Nor was there any consensus about when public health officials, technicians, doctors, police, or other government officials could be forced to come into contact with individuals suspected of being "biologically dangerous." Since these groups did not have to interact with those deemed biologically dangerous by court order except on a voluntary basis, it was difficult to find a legal basis to compel interaction in the face of prior risk.

Is it possible that certain groups of people could find themselves labeled as dangerous to others by dint of their biological makeup? What would be the legacy of current disputes about the duties of health care providers and others to interact with people infected with HIV when advances in genetics allow very precise determinations as to who is and is not likely to transmit disease?

Case 5. Public Health and Good Mating Practices

The newest virtual reality tapes (VRs) on marriage and childbearing from the Minnesota Department of Health and Procreation were ready for distribution.[13] They warned young people about the economic consequences for the state and for themselves of reproducing without a genome test. The public service VRs made a very persuasive case that certain groups known to be at high risk of bringing children into the world with disabling and costly disorders and defects, such as diabetes, gout, deafness, migraines, panic disorders, and allergies, should get a complete genetic analysis before mating and procreating. Strong reinforcement stimuli introducing subliminal messages were used to urge young couples to get an embryo biopsy before sending their offspring off for incubation at the fetal nursery.

Many civil libertarians were aghast at the idea that the state could coerce reproductive behavior. While no one disagreed about the importance of using genetic information to encourage responsible parenting, to many people it seemed wrong for the state to try to compel such behavior. Yet, since there had been no effort to create a right to privacy following the dismantling of *Roe v. Wade* in the mid-2010s, it was almost impossible to find a basis to protect procreative liberty against the interests of the state in protecting the public good. Mandating the provision of information about who was at risk of procreating a child having a problem and the financial consequences of an unfortunate pregnancy outcome seemed the only way to handle ethically the question of individuals and groups at risk of passing on deleterious genes.

When should the state be allowed to encourage or require genetic testing, screening, or counseling? What conditions merit such activities? And what bases will individuals and families have to assert their rights to reproduce in the face of an overwhelming state interest in minimizing the burden of disease and disability on the community?

Case 6. Mass Screening for Bad Blood

The National Health Insurance program announced its intent to create a screening program to detect genetic markers associated with especially high risk for high blood pressure. The burden imposed by illnesses related to high blood pressure, such as diabetes and stroke, was such that the program sought to screen all groups believed to be at higher than average risk for the disorder. Broad screening would permit early intervention using psychological as well as pharmacological methods. But the program had limited funds to carry out screening, counseling, and follow-up interventions. Since it had been established in the 1970s that African-Americans were at especially high risk of high blood pressure,[14] the program intended to make this group the first population targeted for screening and intervention.

The federal insurance program was built on a two-step strategy. The program would provide information on stress management, relaxation, and free medications that could lower blood pressure with only minimal risks of side effects. Higher premiums would be charged to those identified at high risk who failed to manage their blood pressure responsibly.

Would it be ethical to target a particular racial group, whose membership is defined by culture and history, for genetic screening? Should such programs be undertaken if there are penalties attached for noncompliance? What will greater information about the risks created by one's genetic makeup do to our understanding of the concepts of personal responsibility and voluntary choice?

WHAT IS A "RACE" AND WHO ARE ITS MEMBERS?

A number of issues concerning justice, fairness, and equity for minority groups arise from the previous six cases. Emerging knowledge about human heredity will have enormous implications for the use of genetic information to classify human beings and for understanding the reality and legitimacy of racial and ethnic classification schemes, the purposes for which testing and screening are done, the selection of traits to screen, and the need to protect privacy and confidentiality. The extent to which beliefs about heredity and human genetics have been used, abused, and misused in the past indicates how important it is that discussion begin now about the normative and prescriptive stand that is appropriate for shaping social policy in the light of rapidly expanding knowledge of the genome in the future.

Perhaps no question is more pressing from the viewpoint of ethnic and racial minorities than understanding the ways in which new genetic knowledge will shape their self-understanding and social standing. Should knowledge generated by the genome project be used to identify, classify, or label racial or ethnic groups or to establish the boundaries of their membership? When screening programs are undertaken for groups, should the traditional cultural and political definitions of race and ethnicity prevail or will—and to what extent can—biological definitions be used? Will the information generated by the genome project be used to draw new, more "precise" boundaries concerning membership in existing groups? Will individuals who have tried to break their ties with ethnic or racial groups be forced to confront their biological ancestry and lineage in ways that clash with their own self-perception and the lives they have built with others?

It might be argued that it is morally acceptable to use genetic information to classify groups of human beings for scientific purposes, but perhaps not for use solely in the service of social, community, or public policy goals. However, since there may be very real benefits associated with the compilation of information about the medical or psychological needs of certain groups, a better principle might be to avoid testing except when it is undertaken with the goal of benefitting the individual being tested or the group of which that person might be a member. Health professionals in particular will need to be cautious about allowing themselves to be cast into the role of using genetic information for purely social purposes if they hope to retain the trust of minority group members.

While it is possible that the genome project will reveal huge amounts of variation and difference among the genotypes of those persons who are currently lumped together as being in the same ethnic or racial group based upon their phenotypes, it is also likely that some genetic information will be found to be unique or prevalent among the members of certain groups. If this is so, then the temptation to cluster groups in the light of this information may well be unavoidable. Those taking genetic tests may have to be fully informed about the possible threat to self-image and sense of personal identity that this testing may pose. Warnings—genomic informed consent—about the possible impact of genetic testing and screening for individuals in terms of their self-worth, self-esteem, and sense of personal security may have to become commonplace in the not-so-distant future.

Because of the many possible invidious uses of genome profiling, the principles of autonomy and informed voluntary choice will have to be used to regulate the collection and use of genetic information for the purposes of classification. If individuals have a right to their genetic privacy, then new genetic knowledge should not be used to classify those who do not wish to be classified, including children from what we now term "mixed" marriages, potential donors of organs or tissues, or those who for personal reasons do not want their ancestry known to others. Nor should genetic information be used for social policy purposes unless it is shown to be absolutely necessary as a precondition for expanding opportunities or benefits to the members of certain groups and then only if the information is obtained and used with the express permission of the source of the genetic material. The lessons of history count as stern cautions in favor of these broad recommendations. One shudders to think what the use of genetic information based upon the genome might have meant in terms of social policy in Alabama in 1890, Germany in 1939, or South Africa in 1970.

Some attempt must be made to decide what purposes justify genetic screening and the storage of genetic information targeted toward specific racial or ethnic groups. One possible moral stance is that those in biomedical science and health care will not screen groups or populations unless it is for the future benefit of those in the group or other members of the same group. Nontherapeutic testing and screening must be approached with great caution, especially in the light of the historical abuse of genetic information by those responsible for social policies in the past and the potential for abuse that will be possible in the not-so-distant future. Those involved in public health will need to understand their duty to protect the interests, dignity, and rights of individuals against the desire of the community or the state to obtain information that could be used to enact social or financial policies that might be advantageous to many but with a great cost to a few.

The selection of traits, behaviors, and properties to identify, screen, and classify should be driven by a concern to identify what is incapacitating, disabling, or damaging to the members of groups rather than merely what is characteristic, distinctive, or typical of a group. The classification of human beings into groups, races, subgroups, and ethnic groups must be undertaken with great care. The ethics of human systematics that will emerge is likely to become one of the greatest moral challenges to face those involved with the human genome project.

RACE, CLASS, AND GENETICS IN THE HERE AND NOW

The hypothetical case studies raised earlier present obvious challenges to the ways in which new knowledge about heredity will impact public policy, our notions about race, and the ethics of health care. But one need not await new knowledge about genetics to see how information about biological differences influences and shapes the distribution and allocation of resources to the members of racial and minority groups. The allocation of organ and tissue transplants is currently extremely sensitive to the nature of group-based biological differences in ways that raise important questions about the ethics of using emerging genetic information concerning human populations.

Study after study has appeared in recent years showing that access to cadaver kidneys for transplants for those with renal failure does not reflect the actual need for kidney transplants in the general population in the United States.[15] African-Americans are underrepresented relative to the percentage of whites with renal failure who receive transplants. Many explanations have been advanced as to why the difference in rates of kidney transplantation exists between blacks and whites, including differences in the age of onset of renal failure, differences in the type and severity of the illnesses causing renal failure, and socioeconomic differences that are thought to correlate with compliance and thus with the efficacy of kidney transplantation.

However, one key reason for the difference in rates between the races is the reliance of many programs on antigen matching in determining who will have priority for receiving available kidneys.

Certain crucial biological markers have been identified in key components of the immune system—the lymphocytes—that are fairly predictive of whether or not an organ from a particular person will trigger a strong immunological reaction in the recipient. When a cadaver is identified and permission is given to procure a kidney, surgeons remove the kidneys and, if possible, lymph nodes in order to maximize the changes of obtaining a sample of healthy lymphocytes to allow for the identification or "typing" of antigens. Standard classification systems have evolved for categorizing characteristic markers found on well-mapped areas of these antigens. Many transplant surgeons look for the best possible match between donor and recipient on the A, B, and Dr loci even though these are not the only areas governing immunological resistance. By mixing lymphocytes with various known forms of human sera, it is possible to determine the degree of biological similarity between donor and recipient on these important loci.

The reliance on tissue typing is believed by many to correlate with increased changes for successful engraftment in kidney and other forms of transplants.[16] Many studies show that significant differences, between five and ten percent, in outcomes at one year and five years of survival can be shown for kidneys transplanted between donors and recipients who are biologically similar to one another. Full matches at the A, B, and Dr loci, which rarely occur due to the enormous variation that exists among the immune systems of human beings, have such marked success in terms of graft survival that the current national health systems for distributing organs in the United States and Europe mandate that a cadaver kidney always be made available to a recipient who is a full match for it.

In terms of equitable distribution of kidneys among blacks and whites, the use of antigen matching as a critical factor in allocating kidneys means those who are members of minority groups have a lower probability of receiving a transplant. Since the antigens are closely linked to race and ethnicity, it is much easier to find a biological match among people with similar ethnic and racial backgrounds than it is among any two randomly selected individuals. On the basis of tissue matching, organs from blacks will almost always go to blacks and organs from whites will almost always go to whites. Blacks, however, have a much higher incidence of kidney failure than whites. But since whites significantly outnumber blacks in the American population, there are still large numbers of whites waiting for organs. There are so many, in fact, that nearly every white donor is matched to a white recipient. Blacks and other minorities must rely on a much smaller pool of kidneys. The situation for potential black kidney transplant recipients is made even worse by the fact that blacks have a lower rate of cadaver organ donation than do whites. So there is a disproportionately small share of black cadaver kidneys available for a disproportionately large group of blacks in need of kidney transplants. By deciding to use biology in the name of efficiency and, it must be added, fairness, whites wind up with a much larger number of kidney transplants than do blacks relative to the incidence of renal failure in both groups.

The reality of the dilemma that exists between being guided by considerations of efficacy and equity in the allocation of cadaver kidneys for transplantation today is likely to become all too familiar as new knowledge about genetics points the way toward the more efficacious use of medical resources tomorrow. The challenge societies will face is deciding to what extent the values of equal opportunity and fairness justify modifications in policies aimed at the maximization of effectiveness when it is biology that influences the chances for success. Whatever the answer offered in response to situations in which biology points in one direction but notions of equal opportunity and fairness point in another, it is important that the answer be formulated publicly so that those whose interests are at issue can demand accountability from those who must ultimately decide.

NOTES

1. P. Kahn, "Germany's Gene Law Begins to Bite," *Science* 255 (1992): 524–546.

2. See R. J. Lifton, *The Nazi Doctors* (New York: Basic Books, 1986); B. Müller-Hill, *Murderous Science* (New York: Oxford University Press, 1988); R. Proctor, *Racial Hygiene: Medicine under the Nazis* (Cambridge, Mass.: Harvard University Press, 1988); M. H. Kater, *Doctors under Hitler* (Chapel Hill, NC.: University of North Carolina Press, 1989); A. L. Caplan, "The End of a Myth," *Dimensions: A Journal of Holocaust Studies* 5 (1990): 13–18, and A. L.

Caplan, ed., *When Medicine Went Mad: Bioethics and the Holocaust* (Totowa, N.J.: Humana Press, 1992).

3. See M. Biagioli, "Science, Modernity, and the Final Solution," in S. Friedlander, ed., *Probing the Limits of Representation* (Cambridge, Mass.: Harvard University Press, 1992) and Caplan, *When Medicine Went Mad.*

4. See P. Weindling, "Weimar Eugenics: The Kaiser Wilhelm Institute for Anthropology, Human Heredity and Eugenics in Social Context," *Annals of Science* 42 (1985): 303–318; Proctor, *Racial Hygiene;* W. E. Seidelman, "Mengele's Medicus: Medicine's Nazi Heritage," *Milbank Quarterly* 66 (1988): 221–239; C. Pross, "Breaking through the Postwar Coverup of Nazi Doctors in Germany," *Journal of Medical Ethics* 17 (1991): 13–16; Caplan, *When Medicine Went Mad;* R. M. Lerner, *Final Solutions: Biology, Prejudice and Genocide* (University Park, Penn.: Pennsylvania State University Press, 1992).

5. Caplan, *When Medicine Went Mad.*

6. Lifton, *Nazi Doctors;* Proctor, *Racial Hygiene;* Seidelman, "Mengele Medicus"; Kater, *Doctors under Hitler;* Pross, "Breaking through"; Biagioli, "Science"; Caplan, *When Medicine Went Mad;* Lerner, *Final Solutions;* M. Burleigh and W. Wipperman, *The Racial State: Germany 1933–1945* (New York: Cambridge University Press, 1992).

7. Caplan, *When Medicine Went Mad.*

8. Proctor, *Racial Hygiene;* P. Reilly, *The Surgical Solution* (Baltimore: Johns Hopkins University Press, 1991).

9. D. Bergsma, ed., *Ethical, Social and Legal Dimensions of Screening for Human Genetic Disease* (New York: Stratton, 1974).

10. Marc Lappé, *Broken Code* (San Francisco: Sierra Club Books, 1984); T. Duster, *Backdoor to Eugenics* (New York: Routledge, 1990).

11. D. Kumar, "Should One be Free to Choose the Sex of One's Child?" *Journal of Applied Philosophy* 2 (1985): 197–204.

12. P. Applebome, "The Ex-Nazi Who Would be Governor," *New York Times,* 10 November 1991, pp. 1, 17.

13. "Being and Believing: Ethics of Virtual Reality," *Lancet* 338 (1991): 283–284.

14. A. A. Tyroler, S.A. James, "Blood Pressure and Skin Color," *American Journal of Public Health* 68 (1978): 1170–1172; E. Harburg, L. Gleibermann, P. Roeper, M. A. Shork, and W. J. Schull, "Skin Color, Ethnicity and Blood Pressure: Detroit Blacks," *American Journal of Public Health* 68 (1978): 1177–1183.

15. R. P. Kusserow, *The Distribution of Organs for Transplantation: Expectations and Practices* (Washington, D.C.: Government Printing Office, 1990 [OEI-1-89-00550]).

16. E. P. Vichinsky, et al., "Alloimmunization in Sickle Cell Anemia and Transfusion of Racially Unmatched Blood," *New England Journal of Medicine* 322 (1990): 1617–1621.

4

PUBLIC CHOICES AND PRIVATE CHOICES
Legal Regulation of Genetic Testing

Lori B. Andrews

The use of genetic testing by individuals and society is a mixture of private and public choices. Individual conceptions about the importance of a particular health status, disability, prenatal life, and the financial costs or social risks of using genetic testing figure into the individual decision about whether or not to undergo a genetic test. But these individual choices also take place within a context of legal and regulatory policies.

Policies are in effect that act in various ways to *allow, forbid,* or *require* the use of genetic testing. Even when tests are not mandated by law, private institutions such as employers or insurers might require that tests be undertaken or that information from previous testing be disclosed, thus providing a de facto mandate for testing.

RESTRICTIONS ON THE USE OF GENETIC TESTING

Restrictions on the private use of genetic testing can take a variety of forms. They may occur as outright bans or as barriers to the receipt of information about the existence of a particular genetic test. They may occur as barriers to a particular use of the genetic information, such as a ban on abortion. Or they may occur as a result of fiscal barriers that prevent access to the information, the test, or an additional action based on test results.

Bans on Certain Prenatal Testing

In the current legal climate, the use of nonexperimental genetic tests is clearly allowed and often encouraged by law. In fact, with respect to prenatal diagnosis, physicians can be held liable if they do not advise potential parents of the existence of relevant established genetic tests or if they perform such testing inadequately.[1] The gravamen of this cause of action is that people cannot adequately exercise their constitutional right to make reproductive decisions (such as the decision to use contraception or to abort) without sufficient information.[2]

Although prenatal diagnosis via currently established modalities is clearly allowable, state statutes focusing on protecting embryos and fetuses ban certain new modalities for prenatal diagnosis of genetic anomalies. Prime among these restrictions are the state fetal research laws in effect in twenty-four states.[3] In seven states, experimental procedures may not be used on a fetus *in utero* unless they are therapeutic to the fetus or, in some states, unless they pose no discernible risk to the fetus.[4] If the experimental prenatal screening is undertaken to inform the couple's abortion decision, rather than as an initial step toward treatment of the fetus, the procedure would not be considered therapeutic to the fetus. In addition, most *in utero* prenatal diagnostic technologies are interventionist and thus pose a risk of causing miscarriage in a small number of cases. Yet any new form of prenatal diagnosis that is nontherapeutic and poses a risk would be forbidden under the seven restrictive laws.

In addition, under two state statutes, *ex utero* genetic testing on embryos would be forbidden.[5] This would affect the permissibility of embryo biopsy in which a woman's egg is fertilized with a man's sperm in a petri dish. In this procedure, which is still in the research stage, one cell of the embryo is removed and the remaining cells frozen. The single cell is tested for a variety of genetic conditions, such as Down's syndrome. Couples then decide whether they want the embryo implanted.[6]

The use of embryo biopsy is also affected by laws that do not allow embryos to be terminated.[7] Under a Louisiana statute, any human embryo may be used "solely for the support and contribution of the complete development of human in utero implantation."[8] The statute also provides that "A viable in vitro fertilized human ovum is a juridical person which shall not be intentionally destroyed. . . ."[9] Thus, if a couple does learn that their embryo is affected with a defect, the couple would not be able to terminate the embryo. They would have three options: freeze the embryo indefinitely,[10] donate the embryo to another couple who is willing to rear a child with that defect, or have the embryo implanted in the wife and have her undergo a subsequent abortion (since the laws against terminating *in vitro* embryos do not apply after the embryo is reimplanted). Each of these three options present potential financial and emotional costs to the couple that they may not wish to bear.

As new types of prenatal screening tests (such as embryo biopsy) develop, or as old tests (such as amniocentesis) are used in combination with new DNA tests such as that for cystic fibrosis, the benefits of such tests will not be available to couples in states with restrictive laws. Yet such prohibitions interfere with a couple's right to make decisions about reproduction by depriving them of the means of obtaining the information necessary to make that decision. Consequently, such laws could be challenged as being an interference with the couple's right to privacy to make procreative decisions.

In the first case of its kind, *Lifchez v. Hartigan,* a federal district court in Illinois in April 1990 held that the constitutional right to privacy protects a couple's decision to use genetic diagnostic tests on a conceptus, including embryo biopsy.[11] Restrictions on such decisions are unconstitutional unless they further a compelling state interest in the least restrictive manner possible. The court struck down as unconstitutional a law that forbade experimental use of such tests.[12]

In a future case, could a state demonstrate a compelling interest in protecting embryos? Probably not. Its potential interest is not justifiable as an interest in protecting life since the conceptus has not been recognized in law as a person.[13] Rather, it is an interest in protecting the conceptus as a symbol of our high regard for human life. This symbolic protection is also thought to make it more likely that we will treat with appropriate regard certain vulnerable groups in society such as seriously ill newborns, comatose individuals, and elderly patients. The underlying assumption of this view is that the conceptus, though it may not be a person, nevertheless has a special status; it is symbolic of human life or represents life in a way that makes its destruction symbolic of the destruction of persons. Persons who hold this view claim that harm to conceptuses may influence our attitudes toward and treatment of people after birth (particularly comatose people, the elderly, and seriously ill newborns)—that we may come to treat the symbolized no better than we have treated the symbol. The notion is that proscribing procedures that are potentially harmful to conceptuses is a symbolic expression of our interest in human life, an expression that may be necessary for sustaining the level of respect persons deserve.

The protection of symbols is an important part of our legal culture, but it is not sufficient to justify infringing upon a fundamental constitutional right. There is no empirical evidence that actions toward a symbolic entity negatively influence the way actual people are treated.[14] This is particularly true in the case of early embryos, which are undifferentiated cell masses and do not resemble people, so that it is unlikely that actions toward *in vitro* embryos will shape our actions toward newborns, comatose people, elderly patients, or other persons.[15] It would be unconstitutional to ban on symbolic grounds alone the use of experimental techniques on embryos, such as embryo biopsy, that further procreative decisions. However, there may be a sufficient state interest in protecting the conceptus against pain such that a fetal research law restricting experimentation after the fetus could feel pain could be justified.[16]

Some states that do not ban genetic testing nonetheless have adopted statutes that eliminate tort actions against physicians for providing inadequate or inaccurate genetic testing or genetic information.[17] The constitutionality of such statutes must be scrutinized as well, however. A person's right to privacy to make reproductive decisions includes a right to information upon which to make that decision. By not allowing courts to hold physicians liable when they fail to provide that information, states with statutes prohibiting wrongful birth actions eliminate incentives for physicians to disclose such information, thus interfering with the couple's exercise of their right.[18] In an analogous situation, the Fourth Circuit Court of Appeals recognized that when the state provides inaccurate genetic information and an individual subsequently makes reproductive decisions based on that information, the person can sue for violation of his or her constitutional rights.[19]

The purpose of statutes banning wrongful birth or wrongful life cases is to discourage abortion so as to protect the embryo or fetus.

Thus, these statutes also unconstitutionally infringe upon a couple's rights to privacy without advancing a compelling state interest.

Restrictions on Abortion

What about direct restrictions on abortion? Although the U.S. Supreme Court's decisions in *Webster v. Reproductive Health Services*[20] and *Planned Parenthood v. Casey*[21] indicated a greater willingness on the part of the Court to uphold state regulations restricting abortion, the Court has not specifically overruled *Roe v. Wade.*[22] Even if states were, in the wake of *Webster* and *Casey*, to adopt more restrictive abortion laws, it is likely that they would nevertheless permit abortion when the fetus suffers from a serious genetic defect. Polls of the public show that 74% of Americans surveyed approve of abortion in those circumstances.[23] Even prior to *Roe v. Wade*, model abortion laws promulgated by legal[24] and medical groups[25] would have allowed abortions of fetuses with serious genetic defects.[26]

Although it is likely that abortions for genetic reasons would still be allowed under state laws after an overturning of *Roe v. Wade*, such abortions might be restricted to instances of particularly serious disorders (such as Tay–Sachs[27]). State legislatures might ban abortions when the disorder is not rapidly life threatening, for example, when a prenatal test indicates a late onset disorder such as Huntington's disease, when the disorder has a wide variation of expression such as cystic fibrosis, or when the disorder can be treated after birth such as phenylketonuria.[28]

Fiscal Constraints

Legal barriers are not the only, or even the most serious, constraints on access to genetic testing. Fiscal constraints figure prominently since prenatal genetic screening can cost from $500 to $1,000 or more. Embryo biopsy is even more expensive because fertile couples who want to use it will need to pay the costs of *in vitro* fertilization as well, at least $5,000 per attempt. In cases where the genetic test can only be accomplished through linkage studies, the person who wants to use such testing may have to pay for the costs of all the testing done on family members as well. The financial costs of a particular genetic test are not just a matter of free market whim. They, too, may be influenced by policy decisions. For example, the refusal of the federal government to fund research involving *in vitro* fertilization or embryo biopsy means that costs to patients are higher than they would be if clinical fees were supplemented by research funds. Moreover, insurance companies' refusal to fund experimental technologies or those involving *in vitro* fertilization also increase out-of-pocket costs to patients.[29]

The expense of genetic tests prevents many people from using them. Prenatal diagnosis, for example, is mainly used by women from the middle and upper classes.[30] This disparity has implications for public policy far beyond the area of genetic testing per se. Prior to the advent of prenatal diagnosis, a child with a genetically based mental or physical disability could be born into a family of any socioeconomic status. Middle class and wealthier families used resources and connections to lobby state legislatures to pass laws providing for adequate education for children with disabilities.[31] With the use of prenatal diagnosis and abortion, fewer such children are being born to couples of higher socioeconomic status. Affected children may become—like "crack" babies and boarder babies—an issue for the poor, with many fewer protections and resources available to them.

PUBLIC CHOICES

In contrast to the restrictions on private choices in the use of genetic testing, there are potential public pressures in the opposite direction. There are a number of ways in which the state can encourage or mandate the use of genetic testing. It can require a particular test, it can make a person liable in tort for not undertaking the test, or it can allow institutions (such as insurance companies) to condition benefits on submission to the tests. At a more subtle level, it can require that people be informed about the test, provide financial incentives for people to take the test, or even pay for the test directly. To the extent that these public actions interfere with private choices, they need to be justified by strong public interest. The types of public interests usually set forth to justify such actions are the governmental concern for safety and health and protection of the public fisc.

Mandatory Genetic Screening

The United States has already seen two waves of laws devoted to forcing people to use genetic information. The first were mandatory sterilization laws, enacted by state legislators to prevent people with presumably undesirable genes from reproducing on the grounds that the care of the unfit (such as the mentally disabled) was draining society's resources. The second, more recent wave involved mandatory genetic screening for sickle-cell anemia so that people who were carriers of the gene could use the test results to inform their personal reproductive choices.

The first eugenics law, enacted in Indiana in 1907, provided for the involuntary sterilization of institutionalized, unimprovable individuals who were idiots, imbeciles, rapists, or habitual criminals.[32] Eventually, twenty-six other states followed suit,[33] and at least 100,000 people were sterilized under the laws. The Nazi misuse of sterilization did not dampen the American program. In a study of sterilization laws and their implementation, Philip Reilly found that "more than one half of all eugenic sterilizations [in the United States] occurred after the Nazi program was fully operational."[34]

The impetus for the eugenics laws was, in large measure, fiscal. In the 1870s, state governments had provided extensive funding for institutions for the care of the feebleminded, but subsequently they began reassessing this expenditure and decided that the best way to save costs would be to deter the birth of such children in the first place.[35]

In the 1960s and 1970s, however, greater attention to civil rights manifested itself in part through greater judicial protection of reproductive decisions. U.S. Supreme Court cases acknowledged that the government should not intrude into private reproductive decisions.[36] Consequently, many of the mandatory sterilization statutes were repealed.

The focus on civil rights and individual reproductive decisions, however, led to another form of government mandate related to genetics. While the early genetics laws in this country focussed on mandatory sterilization, this more recent form took the approach of mandatory screening. In the early 1970s, some states adopted laws mandating carrier status screening of African-Americans for sickle cell anemia.[37] The idea was that carriers of the disorder may wish to consider that information when making reproductive plans, since if two carriers conceived a child together, there would be a twenty-five percent chance that the child would be affected with sickle cell anemia. This screening program had disastrous consequences.[38] Appropriate counseling was not provided, and people were psychologically harmed by the information. Societal institutions did not know how to use the test results, and consequently, carriers of sickle cell anemia who were themselves healthy were nonetheless discriminated against in insurance and employment.

Although most sickle cell screening laws have been repealed, mandatory genetic screening is currently in effect in limited circumstances. Under an Ohio law, sperm donors must be screened for genetic carrier status for disorders such as Tay–Sachs disease and sickle cell anemia.[39] However, such a provision is not an untoward limitation on the sperm donor since the right to be a genetic parent alone is not as fundamental as the right to be a genetic parent who ultimately rears the child. From the standpoint of the potential rearing parents who wish to use donated semen, they are not involved in an intimate ongoing relationship with the donor where they wish to pass on the donor's personal traits. They view the donated semen in the same way they view a medical treatment; they want it to be safe and effective. In that sense, they expect it to be screened for genetic defects.

But what happens when lawmakers, unschooled in the subtle distinctions between various procreative purposes, start asking, "Why should only the children of sperm donors be healthy?" What happens when they begin passing laws to require screening of potential parents who are procreating coitally? No state laws currently require women to undergo prenatal testing, although commentators have suggested legal sanctions to force people to undergo prenatal diagnosis or to abort fetuses with serious genetic defects.[40] Most likely, lawmakers have not mandated prenatal diagnosis because the currently available techniques of amniocentesis and chorionic villi sampling are invasive and present risk to the pregnant woman[41] and the fetus.[42] However, evolving techniques—such as embryo biopsy for couples already undergoing *in vitro* fertilization or, in the future, maternal blood tests for fetal cells[43]—may be viewed as less risky by legislators, and consequently, laws might be proposed to require such procedures to provide people with information about the genetic status of their fetus. Indeed, researchers working on a prenatal test that could be performed on maternal blood have suggested its suitability for mass screening.[44]

Case law establishes that a competent adult generally has the right to refuse medical care except in limited circumstances—primarily when the person has or is likely to develop a communicable disease that would directly harm others. Even in situations when the state has been recognized to have the power to mandate treatment, the state has been incredibly circumspect in using that power. Vaccinations have been required,[45] but the government generally has not undertaken activities to track down people who might have infections and to keep them from participating in social life or force them to be treated. With respect to AIDS, people have generally not been required to be tested for HIV against their will, although there have been exceptions for individuals accused of certain crimes and for some patients who expose health care workers to possible infection.

Although people may put themselves at risk in decisions regarding medical services, the state has been allowed to intervene when a person has an infectious disease that puts others at risk due to the possibility of contagion. Some commentators argue that mandatory genetic screening is justifiable under communicable disease precedents to prevent people from "transmitting" disease to their offspring. Under the analogy of genetic disease to infectious disease, the government could order interventions on all individuals of reproductive age (since all people carry genetic defects).

The policy concerns raised by attempts to stop the transmission of genetic diseases differ from those addressed to infectious diseases because genetic diseases differentially affect people of different races. Some commentators contest the applicability of the infectious disease model to government actions regarding genetic disorders because "[u]nlike infectious disease which [generally] knows no ethnic, racial, or gender boundaries, genetic disease is the result of heredity," leaving open the possibility for discriminatory governmental actions.[46]

Most reasonable people would be horrified at the thought of forcing people to be sterilized or undergo abortions against their will for eugenic reasons. Upon first consideration, however, they may not be as troubled by mandatory screening for genetic disorders in the absence of forced sterilization or abortion. Some may even argue that mandatory screening, such as carrier testing of people of reproductive age or screening pregnant women's blood to test fetal cells, is not an infringement on procreative rights because it represents at most a modest physical invasion (for example, a blood test) and it merely provides information that the person can use in making decisions about reproduction.

The reason a competent adult has the right to refuse treatment is because each person is entitled to make a choice about the amount of risk he or she is willing to take with respect to medical services. A person may choose to refuse a medical intervention to avoid potential psychological harm, not just potential physical harm. For example, a person may refuse surgery on the grounds that it will be disfiguring. A person may refuse medical intervention on the grounds that it would require too great a change in lifestyle—for example, a particularly athletic person may avoid an intervention because, although potentially beneficial to his or her health, the intervention would limit the individual's physical activities.

It would seem reasonable that people would likewise have the right to refuse mandatory genetic testing as well, even when the screening presents a modest physical intervention (such as a blood test). Genetic testing can result in people obtaining unwanted information, to their psychological detriment. It can result in lifestyle changes, including those precipitated by the release of genetic information to third parties—such as when insurers or employers make adverse decisions against people based on genetic information.

To reach potential childbearers, carrier status screening of adolescents in school, of people of reproductive age generally, or of people applying for marriage licenses has been suggested. However, such screening measures can carry psychological and social risks. In a Montreal Tay–Sachs screening program, several thousand people under age eighteen were screened. The adolescents screened experienced anxiety when they learned they were carriers.[47] In another study, an American adolescent reportedly suffered a psychotic reaction when she was told she was a carrier of Tay–Sachs disease.[48]

Screening of adults, too, can lead to psychological trauma. Some people have committed suicide when they learned they were affected by Huntington's disease. In fact, deaths due to suicide are four times as prevalent among Huntington's disease patients than among the corresponding U.S. Caucasian population.[49] The psychological risks of testing may be why most people at risk for Huntington's disease have not come forward to be tested.

Testing a pregnant woman's blood to learn about the genetic status of her fetus can lead to the woman learning unwanted information about her own genetic status. If, for example, the fetus is affected with a serious recessive genetic disorder, the woman will know that she is a carrier for that disorder. And if a pregnant woman is at risk for a dominant disorder, but has chosen not to undergo genetic testing for that disorder because she does not want to know her genetic status, she may have the unwanted information thrust upon her through a mandatory prenatal blood test. If her fetus has the gene, so does she. In addition to presenting a psychological risk to those individuals who learn that they are carriers or affected by particular genetic disorders, screening can present a psychological risk to those who find they are not carrying the defective gene. According to Nancy Wexler, when at-risk individuals learn that they are not carriers of Huntington's disease, "[m]any may suffer 'survivor guilt,' particularly characteristic of wartime soldiers who live while their buddies are killed."[50]

A National Academy of Science Committee has taken the position that genetic screening should be voluntary.[51] This comports with the individual's right of self-determination and is in keeping with the general legal rule that people have a right to waive information, for example, they can decide to waive the presentation of health care information before they consent to treatment.[52] An individual may not wish to know his or her carrier status.

In addition to its potential detrimental effect on an individual's self-concept, mandatory screening could lead to stigmatization of carriers and potential discrimination.[53] Surveys by Paul Billings and colleagues,[54] as well as by the Office of Technology Assessment of the U.S. Congress,[55] have uncovered examples of people being denied health insurance coverage based on their genotype. These incidents include cases in which a person with a positive test for a genetic disorder had his or her insurance canceled or rated up as a result[56]; where genetic disorders (such as alpha-1-antitrypsin) were defined as preexisting conditions, thus excluding payment for therapy; where a particular genetic condition resulted in exclusion from maternity coverage[57]; and where the birth of a child affected with a serious recessive disorder led to an inability of the parents and unaffected siblings to obtain insurance.[58]

Similar problems exist in the employment context. Twenty-four percent of American geneticists surveyed said they would disclose genetic information to employers, against their patient's wishes.[59] Employers often refuse to hire applicants with any health impairment, even a mild one.[60] A new form of discrimination is occurring in which employers screen to reject candidates (such as diabetics) who are qualified for the job, but who are more likely to use medical benefits programs.[61] Even with respect to disorders in which carrier status leads to little or no ill effects on health (such as sickle cell anemia), discrimination has resulted in the past.[62]

In the reproductive setting, mandatory prenatal screening also interferes with couples' constitutional rights of privacy to make procreative decisions. *Lifchez v. Hartigan* specifically held that the right to privacy covers decisions concerning prenatal genetic testing.[63] Consequently, a mandatory genetic screening law will be upheld as constitutional only if it is necessary to further a compelling state interest in the least restrictive manner possible.

There are two state interests raised to justify mandatory genetic carrier screening or prenatal screening. One is the prevention of harm to third parties; prevention of a genetic defect is analogized to prevention of an infectious disease. The other is the protection of the public fisc by providing information that may prevent the birth of a child with serious mental or physical handicaps.

With respect to other fundamental rights, such as freedom of speech, the government has only been allowed to interfere to protect against a danger that is substantial, imminent, and irreparable.[64] Arguably, that is the sort of danger that the U.S. Supreme Court envisioned when it upheld an emergency mandatory vaccination law[65] at a time when infectious disease presented a substantial threat to the community.

Certain infectious diseases potentially put the society as a whole at immediate risk since the diseases can be transmitted to a large number of people in a short time. The potential victims are existing human beings who may be total strangers to the affected individual. In contrast to infectious disease, the transmission of genetic diseases does not present an immediate threat to society. While infectious disease can cause rapid devastation to a community, the transmission of genetic disease to offspring does not have an immediate detrimental effect, but rather it creates a potential risk for a future generation in society.[66] U.S. Supreme Court cases dealing with fundamental rights have held that harm in the future is not as compelling a state interest as immediate harm.[67]

It is unlikely that the government will be seen as having a legitimate interest in preventing the birth of children who are affected with genetic disorders. Given the current state of development of medical genetics, in which effective treatment for genetic disorders is rare, prenatal screening and diagnosis generally lead to abortion of the affected fetuses.

Because the state could not show that the policy improves the health of potential children, it is likely to have to fall back on the argument that such a policy advances a state interest in saving money. However, a state interest in saving money should not override fundamental rights.[68] Also, it is unclear that the state could prove, in a cost–benefit analysis, that screening actually would save a sufficient amount of money to justify infringement upon individual choice. While aborting a fetus with a particular disorder may represent a savings to society of the cost of rearing that child, it may be that the overall costs of screening and providing necessary counseling and other services for the entire reproductive age population to find carriers or even just of screening prenatally would be so great that it would not offset the costs of rearing the few affected children whose births the state is trying to prevent.

It is likely that no statute actually mandating carrier screening or prenatal screening will ultimately be upheld as constitutional. However, it may be constitutional for the state to adopt a law that mandates that physicians inform pregnant women of the availability of prenatal screening and treatment, which the women could then choose to undergo or refuse. This is the current approach taken in a California program that requires physicians to inform their patients about maternal serum alpha-fetoprotein testing.[69] Another role that the government could play would be the provision of funds to subsidize voluntary prenatal screening and treatment.

Newborn Screening

While the mandating of a genetic test or treatment is generally an extremely rare occurrence, state-sponsored newborn screening programs are in effect in all states for the genetic disorder of phenylketonuria (PKU). Earlier identification of infants with PKU allows a treatment that can dramatically prevent mental retardation. In at least three states (Michigan, Montana, and West Virginia), screening is mandatory without exception.[70] In contrast, the statutes of three jurisdictions (the District of Columbia, Maryland, and North Carolina) clearly provide that newborn screening is voluntary.[71] Other states have provisions allowing parents to refuse the test or the test may be refused on religious grounds,[72] and in nine states, parents may object to the test for any reason.[73] However, parents are seldom told of their right to refuse, and hence, even states that are not technically mandatory operate as if they are. Two states go so far as to provide criminal penalties for parents who refuse to allow their children to undergo newborn screening.[74]

Many states also test for a variety of other disorders, in which early intervention can provide a benefit to the newborn, such as hypothyroidism and sickle cell anemia. However, these de facto mandatory programs are also used in some states to test for disorders when there is no evidence that such a test is necessary. In three states, newborn screening is undertaken for cystic fibrosis even though a double-blind study has shown that early intervention is not necessary since children can be treated with equally good results once they become symptomatic. In some other countries, newborn screening is undertaken for Duchenne muscular dystrophy; since there is no treatment for the affected child, the purpose of the screening is to give the infant's parents information that might be relevant to their future reproductive plans.

It seems inappropriate to mandate a medical intervention on an infant when there is no immediate benefit to that infant. Even when there is a necessary therapy available—such as when the child is affected with PKU—questions can be raised regarding whether mandatory genetic screening is an appropriate policy choice.

In other areas, parents are allowed to refuse medical interventions involving their children. Only when their decisions put their children at grave risk are parental decisions overridden by the state. For example, when parents refuse to allow a blood transfusion to their child, placing the child at risk of serious harm or death, a court will generally order the transfusion over the objections of the parents. However, refusal of a newborn screening test is not analogous to refusal of a blood transfusion. While there is virtual certainty that refusal of the blood transfusion will lead to grave harm to the child, refusal of a newborn screening test is unlikely to harm a particular child. Consider newborn screening for PKU. If the incidence of PKU is 1 in 12,000 to 15,000, the chance is very small indeed that a child who is not screened will actually be affected.[75] The risk is less than the risk of a false negative from the test.[76] Moreover, the small risk of mental retardation from a refused PKU screen is far less than the risks inherent in many other decisions that parents are routinely allowed to make. For example, society allows parents to decide that their children may participate in high school athletics even though there is probably a greater risk that a child will be injured during such activities than that he or she will be affected by a metabolic disorder in the instance when parents refuse screening.

Because, in the rare instance in which an untested child is affected, the injury to that particular child is so devastating, the President's Commission for the Study of Ethical Problems in Medicine and Biomedical Research suggested that screening might be mandated if it appeared that the number of refusals was high and the number of affected, undiagnosed children was high.[77] However, research suggests that even when a newborn screening program is completely voluntary and parents may refuse for any reason, the actual refusal rate is quite low, about 0.05 percent (27 of 50,000 mothers).[78] In addition, since a voluntary program requires the informed consent of parents, the voluntary program adds a check on the procedure. If parents are told about screening and agree to it, but then notice that the screening has not been done, the parents can take action to ensure that the baby is screened. Thus, more infants may actually be screened under a voluntary program than a mandatory one if parents point out when their infants are inadvertently not screened.

Although opponents of voluntary screening assume that fewer infants will be screened under that approach than with mandatory screening, this is not necessarily the case. In a 1979 study, the percentage of newborns screened was calculated for each of twelve states.[79] The two states with the highest percentage of newborns screened (ninety-eight percent) were Maryland, which has a voluntary program, and New Hampshire, which allows parents to refuse screening for any reason. The other ten states, which all have mandatory programs that require all infants to be screened unless the parents can qualify for religious exemption, had lower percentages of newborns screened. In one of these mandatory states, the proportion of newborns screened was only fifty-eight percent. Naturally, any voluntary program needs as its underpinning an adequate procedure for informing parents and obtaining consent. In a study of Maryland's voluntary program, most nurses reported that it required only one to five minutes to inform a mother about newborn screening.[80]

Tort Liability

Mandatory screening is not the only policy approach that pressures people to undergo genetic testing. So could the potential for tort liability. A California case, *Curlender v. Bio-Science Laboratories*,[81] suggested that a child with a genetic defect could bring suit against her parents for not undergoing genetic screenings and aborting her.[82] This is not without precedent. A Michigan court held that a boy had a cause of action against his mother for taking tetracycline during her pregnancy, which gave him brown teeth.[83] Subsequently, the California legislature, as well as the legislatures of five other states, prohibited suits by children claiming the parents should be liable for not aborting them.[84] Statutes prohibiting wrongful life cases against parents further a couple's autonomy in procreative decisions. As the California Supreme Court pointed out in a later case, the purpose of such legislation is "to eliminate any liability or other similar economic pressure which might induce potential parents to abort or decline to conceive a potentially defective child."[85] While a physician breaches a legal and moral duty by not giving competent advice to allow parents to make an informed decision about whether they should continue a pregnancy, parents are exercising a legal right by choosing not to abort.[86] It is also questionable whether there is much to be gained practically by such suits. Since parents usually pay for a child's support, recovery against them rather than against a third party tortfeasor "would just shift family funds (less lawyers' fees and court costs) from one pocket to another."[87]

Conditioning Benefits

An additional policy approach to coerce testing is to allow private institutions to condition benefits on the results of genetic testing. There is no law, for example, that requires an applicant for insurance to undergo testing or to disclose information about previously undertaken tests. However, such testing may be required by the company if the applicant wants to receive insurance. Such required testing cannot be justified on health promotion grounds because the people denied insurance may not be able to afford medical care, and their health will thus be damaged rather than promoted. The only rationale for such a policy is an economic one—that it is unfair to let people purchase insurance when they know in advance that they will be heavy users of care. Yet the potential for adverse selection is only a problem if one accepts the current insurance system as a given, and there is no reason to do that. Insurance is supposed to be a risk-spreading mechanism. But if people are going to be asked to pay a premium based on their actual future medical costs—which might be predictable when genetic testing reveals, for example, that they will later suffer from Huntington's disease—the risk-spreading benefit is lost. Perhaps the availability of genetic testing will make the current form of insurance obsolete, just as it will make some current forms of medical practice obsolete, and new forms of insurance will be found that actually do spread risks.

Currently, insurance companies do have access to a wealth of genetic information. Only a few states' laws prescribe how insurance companies should use genetic information. Two states prohibit denying an individual life insurance[88] or disability insurance[89] or charging a higher premium[90] solely because the individual has a particular genetic anomaly, such as a sickle cell trait. A California statute prohibits discrimination by insurance companies against people who carry a gene that has no adverse effects on the carrier, but which may affect his or her offspring.[91] A related statute prohibits such discrimination by health care service plans.[92]

Under a Wisconsin law,[93] insurers are prohibited from requiring that applicants undergo DNA testing to determine the presence of a genetic disease or disorder or the individual's predisposition for a particular disease or disorder. Nor may insurers ask whether the individual has had a DNA test or what the results of the test were. Insurers are also prohibited from using DNA test results to determine rates or other aspects of coverage.

In the employment context, the American With Disabilities Act (ADA),[94] passed in 1990, may help contain such discrimination since it prohibits preemployment medical examinations and inquiries designed to uncover information about disabilities unless the examination or inquiry is designed to reveal the applicant's ability to perform job-related tasks.[95] The ADA also prohibits discrimination against individuals with disabilities in any terms, conditions, or privileges of employment. However, the ADA does not prohibit discrimination against carriers. In addition, it is not clear whether a person with an increased risk of genetic disease, but not a definitive diagnosis that he or she will get the disease, will be viewed as having a disability. A deputy legal counsel of the Equal Employment Opportunity Commission has stated that "characteristic predisposition to illness or disease" is not an impairment. "Consequently, the ADA does not protect individuals, who are not otherwise impaired, from discrimination based on genotype alone."[96]

Because of the sickle cell debacle[97] in the early 1970s, a few states have specifically adopted statutes to prohibit mandatory sickle cell screenings as a condition of employment,[98] to prohibit discrimination in employment against people with the sickle cell trait,[99] and to prohibit discrimination by unions against people with the sickle cell trait.[100]

A broader New Jersey law prohibits employment discrimination based on an "atypical hereditary cellular or blood trait."[101] In New York, a statute prohibits genetic discrimination based on the sickle cell trait, Tay–Sachs trait, or the Cooley's anemia (beta-thalassemia) trait.[102] In Oregon, Wisconsin, and Iowa even more comprehensive laws prohibit genetic screening as a condition of employment.[103]

CONCLUSIONS

The dichotomy between public choices and private choices is not as clear as we might like. The "public" choice to mandate carrier status or prenatal screening obviously affects very private choices regarding reproduction. Similarly, a private decision to use carrier or prenatal testing has public ramifications beyond that individual couple or family. If only wealthier people tend to use screening, the current disparity between poor children and rich children will be underscored biologically as well as socially.

This is not to say that private choices in the genetic realm should be prohibited. That would not be a sound policy, nor even a constitutionally permissible course. But it does point out the need to provide additional protections—not just geared to the use of genetic

testing but also to the wide-ranging effects those uses will have. It also
cautions us that any given choice about genetic testing is not just one
single decision but a series of decisions—with which all of us must
live.

NOTES

1. For a review of the cases, see Lori B. Andrews, "Torts and the Double
Helix: Malpractice Liability for Failure to Warn of Genetic Risks," *U. Houston
L. Rev.* 29 (1992): 149–184, 135–158.

2. Ibid. There is evidence that, when faced with the information that their
fetus will have a serious disorder, most potential parents choose to abort. In
a large-scale study of 3,000 amniocenteses, in which 113 fetuses were found
to have chromosomal or biochemical abnormalities, 93.8 percent chose
abortion. M. S. Golbus, W. D. Loughman, C. J. Epstein, G. Halbasch, J. D.
Stephens, and B. D. Hall, "Prenatal Genetic Diagnosis in 3,000 Amniocenteses," *New England Journal of Medicine* 300 (1979): 157–163, 160. In a subsequent study of 7,000 pregnancies in which 149 cytogenic abnormalities
were detected, nearly all women with severely abnormal fetuses elected to
terminate their pregnancies, while only sixty-two percent with a prenatally
diagnosed sex chromosome abnormality did so. Peter A. Benn, Lillian Y. F.
Hsu, Ann Carlson, and Hody L. Tannenbaum, "The Centralized Prenatal
Genetics Screening Program of New York City III: The First 7,000 Cases,"
American Journal of Medical Genetics 20 (1985): 369-384, 369–370.

3. For information about the scope of the fetal experimentation statutes,
see Lori B. Andrews, "Regulation of Experimentation on the Unborn," *Journal of Legal Medicine* 14 (1993): 25–56.

4. *Fla. Stat. Ann.* §390.001(6) (West 1986); *Me. Rev. Stat. Ann.* tit. 22,
§1593 (1992); *Minn. Stat. Ann.* §145.422(1), (2) (West 1989); *Mo. Ann. Stat.*
§188.037 (Vernon 1983); *N.M. Stat. Ann.* §24-9A-4, -5 (1991); *Okla. Stat. Ann.*
tit. 63, §1-735 (West 1984); 18 *Pa. Cons. Stat. Ann.* §3216(a) (Purdon Supp.
1992). Certain of these laws would not apply to genetic screening of embryos
because they deal with older fetuses. The New Mexico statute applies only
to fetuses with a heartbeat or other specified vital signs. *N.M. Stat. Ann.* §24-
9A-1(H) (1991). Because a heartbeat is discernible as early as four weeks,
however, such a statute could apply to experimental variations on chorionic
villi sampling. This statute applies only to formal clinical research programs.

5. *La. Rev. Stat. Ann.* §9:121 *et seq.* (West 1991); *Me. Rev. Stat. Ann.* tit. 22
§1593 (1980). But see *Lifchez v. Hartigan,* 735 F. Supp. 1361 (N.D. Ill.), *aff'd.,*
915 F.2d 260 (7th Cir. 1990), *cert. denied sub. nom., Scholberg v. Lifchez,* 498
U.S. 1069, 111 S.Ct. 787 (1991), which held that such a statute is unconsti-

tutional when applied to genetic screening. Some states specifically exempt genetic screening from their bans on embryo and fetal research. In three other states that ban embryo experimentation, there is an exception for diagnostic procedures. *Mass. Ann. Laws* ch. 112 §12J (Law. Co-op. 1985); *N.D. Cent. Code* §14-02.2-01(2) (1991); *R.I. Gen. Laws* §11-54-1(b) (Supp. 1991).

6. At the eight-cell stage, all cells are totipotent and thus the embryo would develop normally, with no damage attributable to the removal of the one cell. For a description of the benefits of genetic screening of the embryo, see, Cliff Grobstein, *From Chance to Purpose: An Appraisal of External Human Fertilization* (Reading, Mass.: Addison-Wesley, 1981), 123.

7. See, e.g., *La. Rev. Stat.* §9:121 *et seq.* (West 1991).

8. *La. Rev. Stat.* §9:122 (West 1991).

9. *La. Rev. Stat.* §9:129 (West 1991).

10. Freezing the embryo indefinitely might lead to the embryo becoming nonviable, but such an effect would not seem to be the sort of intentional destruction that the statute forbids.

11. *Lifchez v. Hartigan*, 735 F. Supp. 1361, 1376 (N.D. Ill.) *aff'd.*, 915 F.2d 260 (7th Cir. 1990), *cert. denied sub. nom., Scholberg v. Lifchez*, 498 U.S. 1069, 111 S.Ct. 787 (1991).

12. The law was also declared to be unconstitutionally vague. Ibid., 1376.

13. Under the common law, an embryo traditionally was not considered to have the rights of a person. In *Roe v. Wade*, the U.S. Supreme Court scanned the Constitution, looking for provisions with the word "person," and found that none of the contexts "has any possible prenatal application." 410 U.S. 113, 157–158 (1973).

14. As Joel Feinberg notes, the weakness of the symbolic argument is "the difficulty of showing that the alleged coarsening effects really do transfer from primary to secondary objects." Joel Feinberg, "The Mistreatment of Dead Bodies," *Hastings Center Report* 15 (1985): 31–37; 37. He observes that "[w]e can deliberately inhibit sentiment toward one class of objects when we believe it might otherwise motivate inappropriate conduct, yet give it free rein toward another class of objects where there is no such danger." Id. (footnote omitted).

15. Sissela Bok, in arguing for an examination of the reasons for protecting life, argues that we cannot simply equate killing an embryo with murder. "[T]he reasons for protecting life fail to apply here. This group of cells cannot feel the anguish or pain connected with death. Its experiencing of life has not yet begun; it is not yet conscious of the interruption of life nor of the loss of anything it has come to value in life. Nor is it tied by bonds of affection to others." Sissela Bok, "Fetal Research and the Value of Life," in *National Commission for the Protection of Human Subjects of Biomedical and Behavioral Research,* Appendix: Research on the Fetus (1975), 2-1, 2-7. See

also Sissela Bok, "Ethical Problems of Abortion," *Hastings Center Studies* 2 (1974): 32–36; 33.

16. In addition, granting various protections to embryos in a way that does not infringe procreative rights (for example, by allowing suits on the embryo's behalf against third party tortfeasors) would be arguably constitutional. Without a fundamental right at issue, the legislation would be considered constitutional if it was rationally related to a permissible governmental purpose, and the protection of the embryo as a symbol would likely meet that standard.

17. At least four states have statutes that prohibit parents from bringing wrongful birth suits against health care practitioners and institutions. *Minn. Stat. Ann.* §145.424(2) (West 1989); *Mo. Ann. Stat.* §188.130–131 (Vernon Supp. 1992); 42 *Pa. Cons. Stat. Ann.* §8305 (Purdon Supp. 1992) (this statute does not prohibit cases based on intentional misrepresentation); *S.D. Codified Laws Ann.* §21-55-2 (1987). At least eight states prohibit children from bringing wrongful life suits. *Idaho Code* §5-334 (1990); *Ind. Code Ann.* §34-1-1-11 (West Supp. 1992); *Minn. Stat. Ann.* §145.424(1) (West 1989); *Mo. Ann. Stat.* §188.130-1 (Vernon Supp. 1992); *N.D. Cent. Code* §32-03-43 (Supp. 1991); 42 *Pa. Cons. Stat. Ann.* §8305 (Purdon Supp. 1992); *S.D. Codified Laws* §21-55-1 (1987); and *Utah Code Ann.* §78-11-24 (1992).

18. The wrongful birth cases specifically recognize that they are creating an incentive for physicians to provide genetic testing and information. See, e.g., *Berman v. Allen,* 80 N.J. 421, 432, 404 A.2d 8, 14 (1979). *Siemieniec v. Lutheran General Hospital,* 134 Ill. App. 3d 823, 480 N.E. 2d 1227, 1232 (1985).

19. *Avery v. County of Burke,* 600 F.2d 111 (4th Cir. 1981). In that case, a young pregnant woman was erroneously diagnosed by a county health department prenatal clinic as having the sickle cell trait and told that she should undergo sterilization. The health care professionals at the clinic apparently overstated the complications of having the sickle cell trait, telling her that it made her more susceptible to numerous diseases while pregnant, that it made childbirth incredibly dangerous, and that it rendered her unable to take birth control pills. Ibid., 113. She underwent the sterilization, then discovered she did not have the trait. The court held that she had a valid cause of action against the clinic for violation of her constitutional rights for wrongfully causing her sterilization.

20. 492 U.S. 490 (1989).

21. 505 U.S.——, 112 S.Ct. 2791, 120 L. Ed. 2d 674 (1992).

22. The Supreme Court in *Webster* noted that the facts in that case differed from those in *Roe,* giving the Court "no occasion to revisit the holding of *Roe.*" *Webster v. Reproductive Health Services,* 492 U.S. 490 (1989). In *Casey,* the Supreme Court expressly affirmed *Roe,* but rejected the trimester framework, thus reinterpreting the scope of *Roe. Planned Parenthood v. Casey,* 505 U.S.——, 112 S.Ct. 2791 (1992).

23. *National Journal* 21 (1989): 1264.

24. "No-Fault Divorce Act and 'Nonarrest' Custody Bill Are Opposed by the House of Delegates in New Orleans," *American Bar Association Journal* 58 (1972): 379–389, p. 380 (allowing abortion if the physician has reasonable cause to believe "that the child would be born with grave physical or mental defect").

25. American Medical Association, *Proceedings of the AMA House of Delegates* (1967): 40–51 (allowing abortions if there is "documented medical evidence" that the child "may be born with incapacitating physical deformity or mental deficiency").

26. See *Roe v. Wade,* 410 U.S. 113, 141–146 (1973), for a discussion of existing and proposed laws prior to the decision.

27. Tay–Sachs disease is a recessive gene disorder most common in families of Eastern European Jewish origin. Children who have the disease exhibit early progressive and profound retardation, blindness, and paralysis with characteristic cherry red spots on the retina. Death usually occurs by age three or four. *Lawyers' Medical Cyclopedia* § 4.10, 3d ed. (1981).

28. Lori B. Andrews, *Medical Genetics: A Legal Frontier* (Chicago: American Bar Foundation, 1987), 238.

29. Statutes in Arkansas, Hawaii, Illinois, Maryland, Massachusetts, and Rhode Island require insurance companies to pay for *in vitro* fertilization, but these deal with uses for treating infertility rather than for genetic screening purposes.

30. Golbus et al., "Prenatal Genetic Diagnosis," 158. In New York State, this disparity has been addressed through a policy of state funding of amniocentesis for poor women.

31. This is not to say that poorer families did not participate in these efforts but rather that the effort was, in some senses, easier for wealthier families.

32. Philip Reilly, "Eugenic Sterilization in the United States," in A. Milunsky and G. Annas, eds., *Genetics and the Law III* (New York: Plenum, 1985), 230.

33. Ruth Macklin and Willard Gaylin, *Mental Retardation and Sterilization: A Problem of Competency and Paternalism* (New York: Plenum, 1981), 65.

34. Reilly, "Eugenic Sterilization," 235. An official of the American Eugenics Society told the media that the German sterilization plan "showed great courage and statesmanship." Daniel Kevles, *In the Name of Eugenics: Genetics and the Uses of Human Heredity* (New York: Knopf, 1985), 118.

35. Reilly, "Eugenic Sterilization," 230.

36. *Griswold v. Connecticut,* 381 U.S. 479 (1965); *Roe v. Wade,* 410, U.S. 113 (1973).

37. Philip Reilly, *Genetics, Law, and Social Policy* (Cambridge, Mass.: Harvard University Press, 1977), 62–86.

38. Ibid., 67.

39. *Ohio Rev. Code Ann.* §3111.33 (Baldwin 1988).

40. See, e.g., Margery W. Shaw, "Conditional Prospective Rights of the Fetus," *Journal of Legal Medicine* 5 (1984): 63–116. Also see "Constitutional Limitations on State Intervention in Prenatal Care, *Virginia Law Review* 67 (1981): 1051–1067; 1051, 1052.

41. The primary risk is infection. Lori B. Andrews, *New Conceptions: A Consumer's Guide to the Newest Infertility Treatments Including in Vitro Fertilization, Artificial Insemination, and Surrogate Motherhood* (New York: Ballantine, 1985), 59.

42. Ibid., 69. Amniocentesis presents a 1 in 200 risk of fetal death. Chorionic villi sampling presents a two to three percent risk of fetal death. Office of Technology Assessment, U.S. Congress, *Human Gene Therapy—Background Paper*, Appendix A (1984), 65.

43. U. M. Mueller, C. S. Hanes, A. E. Wright, A. Petropoulos, E. DeBoni, F. A. Firgaira, A. A. Morley, D. R. Turner, and W. R. Jones, "Isolation of Fetal Trophoblast Cells From Peripheral Blood of Pregnant Women," *Lancet* 336 (1990): 197–200.

44. According to the researchers, "because the FACS procedure requires sampling of maternal blood rather than amniotic fluid, it could make widespread screening in younger women feasible. . . . Widespread screening is desirable because the relatively large number of pregnancies in women below 35 years old means that they bear the majority of children with chromosomal abnormalities despite the relatively low risk of such abnormalities in pregnancies in this age group." L. A. Herzenberg, D. W. Bianchi, J. Schroder, H. M. Cann, and G. M. Iverson, "Fetal Cells in the Blood of Pregnant Women: Detection and Enrichment by Fluorescence-Activated Cell Sorting," *Proceedings of the National Academy of Science* 76 (1979): 1453–1455, p. 1455.

45. *Jacobson v. Massachusetts*, 197 U.S. 11 (1905).

46. C. Damme, "Controlling Genetic Disease Through Law," *University of California Davis Law Review* 15 (1982): 801–807, p. 807.

47. M. Goodman and L. Goodman, "The Overselling of Genetic Anxiety," *Hastings Center Report* 12 (1982): 20–27, p. 24, citing Clow and Scrivner, "The Adolescent Copes with Genetic Screening: A Study of Tay–Sachs Screening Among High School Students," in M. Kabach, *Tay–Sachs Disease: Screening and Prevention* (New York: A. R. Liss, 1977), 381–393.

48. J. T. R. Clark, "Screening for Carriers of Tay–Sachs Disease: Two Approaches," *Canadian Medical Association Journal* 119 (1978): 549–550, p. 550.

49. L. A. Farrer, "Suicide and Attempted Suicide in Huntington Disease: Implications For Pre-clinical Testing of Persons at Risk," *American Journal of Medical Genetics* 24 (1986): 305–311.

50. Nancy S. Wexler, "A Genetic Jeopardy and the New Clairvoyance," *Progress in Medical Genetics* 6 (1985): 277–304; 298.

51. "Participation in a genetic screening program should not be made mandatory by law, but should be left to the discretion of the person tested, or, if a minor, of the parents or legal guardian." Committee for the Study of Inborn Errors of Metabolism, Division of Medical Sciences, Assembly of Life Sciences, National Research Council, "Recommendations" in *Genetic Screening: Programs, Principles, and Research* (1975), 1, 4.

52. Lori B. Andrews, "Informed Consent Statutes and the Decisionmaking Process," *Journal of Legal Medicine* 5 (1984): 163–217, pp. 215–216. In the reproductive context, earlier U.S. Supreme Court cases involving abortion provided particularly strong protection against governmental actions that required people to receive information since information in the context of reproductive decisions can coerce an individual to make a particular decision. *City of Akron v. Akron Center for Reproductive Health*, 462, U.S. 416, 445 (1993); *Thornburgh v. American College of Obstetricians and Gynecologists*, 476 U.S. 747. However, the recent U.S. Supreme Court case, *Planned Parenthood v. Casey*, 505 U.S.——, 112 S.Ct. 2791, 120 L.Ed. 2d 674 (1992), may have overruled this aspect of *Akron* and *Thornburgh*. The three Justices who wrote the Joint Opinion in *Casey* expressly overruled *Akron* and *Thornburgh* to the extent that those cases "find a constitutional violation when the government requires . . . the giving of truthful, nonmisleading information about the nature of the [abortion] procedure, the attendant health risks and those of childbirth, and the 'probable gestational age' of the fetus" (p. 718). The three Justices stated that *Akron* and *Thornburgh* had gone too far in that respect and were "inconsistent with *Roe*'s acknowledgment of an important interest in potential life," namely, the state's legitimate goal of protecting fetal life (pp. 718–719).

Because the two concurring Justices did not join in this part of the Opinion, the Joint Opinion relies on the conclusions of the four dissenting Justices to reach the required majority (pp. 717–718). When Justice Rehnquist's dissent discusses *Thornburgh* in the context of informed consent, however, it does not join in the overruling of these cases. Instead, Rehnquist simply states that *Thornburgh* is not controlling (p. 775) (Rehnquist, J., dissenting). Rehnquist acknowledges that the Joint Opinion expressly overrules *Akron* and *Thornburgh*, in part, under the "undue burden" standard of review adopted there, but then points out that this standard does not enjoy the majority support of the Court (pp. 765, 772). It does not enjoy the support of the four dissenting Justices.

The effect of the Plurality Opinion in *Casey* is that the Pennsylvania abortion statute's informed consent requirements were upheld despite the rulings of *Akron* and *Thornburgh*. Whether this constitutes an overruling of those cases is unclear. Even if the Joint Opinion legitimately overrules the informed consent portion of *Akron* and *Thornburgh*, its language is narrowly drawn. Thus, its application to other cases and different fact patterns, such as mandatory screening for genetic disorders, may be inappropriate or ineffectual (1986).

53. Wexler, "Genetic Jeopardy," 295.

54. See, e.g., P. R. Billings, M. A. Kohn, M. de Cuevas, J. Beckwith, J. S. Alper, and M. R. Natowicz, "Discrimination as a Consequence of Genetic Testing," *American Journal of Human Genetics* 50 (1992): 476–482.

55. U.S. Congress, Office of Technology Assessment, *Cystic Fibrosis and DNA Tests: Implications of Carrier Screening* (August 1992), 200.

56. The disorders included adult polycystic kidney disease, Huntington's disease, neurofibromatosis, Marfan's syndrome, Down's syndrome, and Fabray's disease.

57. The conditions included a balanced translocation.

58. The disorder was cystic fibrosis.

59. Dorothy Wertz and John C. Fletcher, *Ethics and Human Genetics: A Cross-Cultural Perspective* (New York: Springer-Verlag, 1989), 440.

60. Murray Weinstock and Jacob I. Haft, "The Effect of Illness on Employment Opportunities," *Archives of Environmental Health* 29 (1974): 79–83; 83. ("The results of this study suggest that in the area sampled, even patients with mild illnesses, which may not increase their morbidity or mortality, are being denied work").

61. M. Baram, "Charting the Future Course for Corporate Management of Genetics and other Health Risks," in A. Milunsky and G. Annas, eds., *Genetics and the Law III* (New York: Plenum, 1985), 475, 480.

62. James Bowman, "Identification and Stigma in the Workplace," in J. Weiss, B. Bernhardt, and N. Paul, eds., "Genetic Disorders and Birth Defects in Families and Society: Toward Interdisciplinary Understanding," *Birth Defects Original Article Series 20* (1984): 223–225; 225.

63. *Lifchez v. Hartigan*, 735 F. Supp. 1361 (N.D. Ill.), *aff'd.*, 915 F.2d 260 (7th Cir. 1990), *cert. denied sub. nom.*, *Scholberg v. Lifchez*, 498 U.S. 1069, 111 S.Ct. 787 (1991).

64. For example, in *New York Times v. United States*, 403 U.S. 713 (1971), the U.S. Supreme Court, in a per curium opinion held that the government had not met its "heavy burden" of proving that national security required that the Pentagon Papers be suppressed. The logic of the case was explained further in the concurrences; the right of free speech is to be infringed by a prior restraint only when disclosure "will surely result in direct, immediate, and irreparable damage to our Nation or its people" (p. 730) (Stewart, J., concurring) or when there is "governmental allegation and proof that publication must inevitably, directly, and immediately cause the occurrence of

an event kindred to imperiling the safety of a transport already at sea . . ."
during wartime (pp. 726–727) (Brennan, J., concurring).

The standard of irreparability for granting an injunction against protected speech is an absolute, not a comparative, standard. Even if the speech could cause great harm, that would not be sufficient. As Justice White pointed out in his concurrence in *New York Times*, it is not sufficient that there may be "substantial damage to public interests" (p. 731) (White, J., concurring.) Similarly, Justice Stewart said "I am convinced that the Executive is correct with respect to some of the documents involved [i.e., they should not, in the national interest be published]. But I cannot say that disclosure of any of them will surely result in direct, immediate, and irreparable harm to our Nation or its people. That being so, there can under the First Amendment be but one judicial resolution of the issue before us" (p. 730) (White, J., concurring).

Even if irreparable harm were a possibility, *New York Times* indicates that an injunction should not be issued against the press unless such harm would come about directly and immediately. The term *immediately* is easy enough to understand; it requires a present, not future, harm. The term *directly* relates to the lack of intervening influences during that time period. The irreparable harm would not occur directly if another important influence would or could intervene. Another way of expressing the immediacy and directness that is necessary is by saying the harm is *inevitable*—it will occur within a short period of time during which nothing will or could change it or stop it.

Even when a prior restraint is not at issue, high standards are required for showing a compelling state interest when a fundamental right is at issue. Also in the First Amendment area, speech that is not false should not be the basis for subsequent punishment unless it provided an immediate threat of serious harm. (See, e.g., *Bridges v. California*, 314 U.S. 252, 263 (1941); "the substantial evil must be extremely serious and the degree of imminence extremely high before utterances can be punished").

65. *Jacobson v. Massachusetts*, 197 U.S. 11 (1905).

66. Moreover, it should be noted that this risk (transmission of genetic disease to offspring) is one that society has always lived with and seems to have flourished despite that risk.

67. See, e.g., the discussion of *New York Times v. United States* in note 64.

68. In U.S. Supreme Court cases, the goal of protecting the public treasury has not been found to be superior to protecting individual rights. A person's right to travel is recognized as more important than the drain on the welfare system of the state to which he moves. See, e.g., *Edwards v. California*, 314 U.S. 160 (1941). Due to a person's fundamental right of privacy to make procreative decisions, a state may not condition welfare on an in-

dividual's cessation of childbearing. "People are free to move and to be burdens on the state, and procreate and be burdens with their children on the state. If the consequence of a protected act means direct state support, that is the unpredictable price a free society has to pay." Jonathan A. Weiss and Stephen B. Wizner, "Pot, Prayer, Politics, and Privacy: The Right To Cut Your Own Throat in Your Own Way," *Iowa Law Review* 54 (1969): 709–735, pp. 733–734. Weiss and Wizner point out that the government in other ways uses its finances to support choice in the area of constitutional freedom: "Armies are raised and supported so that people may live freely. The consequent loss of income and burden on the state are the price of supporting freedoms of choice" (p. 734, n. 113). Thus, there are valid policy reasons for not holding potential economic costs as a sufficiently compelling governmental interest to outweigh the privacy right to make reproductive decisions.

69. See, e.g., Robert Steinbrook, "In California, Voluntary Mass Prenatal Screening," *Hastings Center Report* 16 (1986): 5–8; 5; 17 Calif. Code of Administrative Regulations 6527 (1992).

70. *Mich. Comp. Laws Ann.* §333.5431 (West 1992); *Mont. Code Ann.* §50-19-203 (1991); *W. Va. Code* §16-22-3 (Miche Supp. 1992).

71. Andrews, *Medical Genetics*, 238.

72. Ibid., citing laws in Alabama (1984), California, Connecticut, Georgia, Hawaii, Idaho, Illinois, Indiana, Kansas, Kentucky, Massachusetts, Minnesota, Mississippi, Missouri, Nebraska, New Jersey, New York, North Dakota, Ohio, Oklahoma, Oregon, Pennsylvania, Rhode Island, South Carolina, South Dakota, Tennessee, Texas, Utah, Virginia, Washington, and Wisconsin. In another state, the law empowers an agency to determine whether testing should be mandatory. In Maine, the Department of Human Services is authorized to make the program mandatory, but provision for religious objection is made.

73. Ibid., citing laws in Alaska, Arizona, Colorado, Florida, Louisiana, Nevada, New Hampshire, New Mexico, and Wyoming.

74. *Mo. Ann. Stat.* §191.331(5) (Vernon 1990); *S.C. Code* §44-37-30(B) (1991).

75. Delbert A. Fisher, Barbara L. Foley, and Marvin Mitchell, "Problems and Pitfalls of Newborn Screening Programs Based on the Experience in California and New England," in Lori B. Andrews, ed., *Legal Liability and Quality Assurance in Newborn Screening* (Chicago: American Bar Foundation, 1985), 38, 39.

76. Delbert Fisher presentation, Conference on Legal Liability in Newborn Screening, American Bar Foundation (15–16 October 1984).

77. *President's Commission for the Study of Ethical Problems in Medicine and Biomedical and Behavioral Research, Screening and Counseling for Genetic Condi-*

tions: The Ethical, Social, and Legal Implications of Genetic Screening, Counseling, and Education Programs (Washington, D.C.: U.S. Government Printing Office, 1983), 6.

78. Ruth Faden, A. Judith Chwalow, Neil A. Holtzman, and Susan D. Horn, "A Survey to Evaluate Parental Consent As Public Policy for Neonatal Screening," *American Journal of Public Health* 72 (1982): 1347–1352, p. 1350.

79. Stephen Sepe, Harvey Levy, and Frank Mount, "An Evaluation of Routine Follow-Up Blood Screening of Infants for Phenylketonuria," *New England Journal of Medicine* 300 (1979): 606. See Andrews, *Medical Genetics,* for an analysis of the voluntary or mandatory nature of screening in each state.

80. Faden et al., "Survey to Evaluate," 1350.

81. 106 Cal. App. 3d 811, 829, 165 Cal. Rptr. 477 (2d Dist. 1980).

82. Subsequently, California and five other states adopted statutes eliminating such a cause of action. *Cal. Civ. Code* §43.6 (West 1982); *Idaho Code* §5-334 (1990); *Minn. Stat. Ann.* §145.424(1) (West 1989); *N.D. Cent. Code* §32-03-43 (Supp. 1991); *S.D. Codified Laws* §21-55-1 (1987); and *Utah Code Ann.* §78-11-24 (1992).

83. *Grodin v. Grodin,* 102 Mich. App. 396, 301 N.W.2d 869 (1980).

84. *Cal. Civ. Code* §43.6 (West 1982); *Idaho Code* §5-334 (1990); *Minn. Stat. Ann.* §145.424(1) (West 1989); *N.D. Cent. Code* §32-03-43 (Supp. 1991); *S.D. Codified Laws* §21-55-1 (1987); *Utah Code Ann.* §78-11-24 (1992).

85. *Turpin v. Sortini,* 31 Cal. 3d 220, 643 P.2d 954, 959, 182 Cal. Rptr. 337 (1982).

86. Alexander Capron, "Legal Rights and Moral Rights," in B. Hilton, D. Callahan, M. Harris, P. Condliffe, and B. Berkeley, eds., *Ethical Issues in Human Genetics: Genetic Counseling and The Use of Genetic Knowledge* (Fogarty International Proceedings No. 13, 1973), 221, 237.

87. Ibid., at 236.

88. *Fla. Stat. Ann.* §626.9706(1) (West 1984); *La. Rev. Stat. Ann.* §22:652.1(D) (West Supp. 1992).

89. *Fla. Stat. Ann.* §626.9707(1) (West 1984); *La. Rev. Stat. Ann.* §22:652.1(D) (West Supp. 1992).

90. *Fla. Stat. Ann.* §626.9076(2) (West 1984) (life insurance); §626.9707(2) (West 1984) (disability insurance); *La. Rev. Stat. Ann.* §22:652.1(D) (West Supp. 1992).

91. *Cal. Ins. Code* §10143 (West Supp. 1992).

92. *Cal. Health & Safety Code* §1374.7 (West 1990).

93. *1991 Wisc. Act 269,* codified as *Wisc. Stat. Ann.* §631.89.

94. 104 Stat. 327 (1991), 42 *U.S.C.A.* §12101 *et seq.* (Supp. 1992).

95. 42 *U.S.C.A.* §12112(4)(A) (Supp. 1992).

96. Letter by Elizabeth M. Thorton, Deputy Legal Director, U.S. Equal

Employment Opportunity Commission to Drs. Paul Berg and Sheldon Wolff, Co-Chairmen, NIH-DOE Joint Subcommittee on the Human Genome, 2 August 1991.

97. Andrews, *Medical Genetics,* 18.

98. This same law appears in three places in the Florida statutes: *Fla. Stat. Ann.* §448.076 (West 1981); §228.201 (West 1989); and §63.043 (West 1985).

99. *Fla. Stat. Ann.* §448.075 (West 1981); *N.C. Gen. Stat.* §95-28.1 (1989); *La. Rev. Stat. Ann.* §23:1002(A)(1) (West 1985).

100. *La. Rev. Stat. Ann.* §23:1002(C)(1) (West 1985).

101. *N.J. Stat. Ann.* §10:5-12(a) (West Supp. 1992).

102. *N.Y. Civ. Rights Law* §48 (McKinney 1992).

103. *Iowa Code Ann.* §729.6 (West 1992); *Wis. Stat.* §111.372 (1991–1992).

5

RULES FOR GENE BANKS
Protecting Privacy in the Genetics Age

George J. Annas

Medical information is becoming less protected and private in the United States. Biographer Diane Wood Middlebrook, for example, was supplied with 300 audiotapes of sessions Anne Sexton had with her psychiatrist, Martin Orne. Dr. Orne not only thought it was ethically acceptable to breach his patient's confidentiality in this way, he himself wrote the forward to the biography that begins with a description of "my first therapy session with Anne Sexton."[1] Although he contends Anne Sexton would have consented to the release of her medical records, she never did during her lifetime and in fact released only four of the tapes to the University of Texas which holds her papers.

Similarly, two days after Earvin "Magic" Johnson announced that he was infected with HIV, the physician who did the confirmatory blood work in New York released confidential medical information about Magic to *New York Times* reporter (and physician) Lawrence Altman, which was printed without any comment on the violation of privacy and confidentiality involved.[2] Four months later, when Altman wrote a front-page story in the *New York Times* about Presidential candidate Paul Tsongas's treatment for cancer and prospects for continued health, he made it clear that Tsongas himself had authorized his physicians to discuss the details of his treatment and current state of health.[3]

Presidents and presidential candidates seem to have accepted the reality that they cannot claim the privacy of the average American. But the privacy of average Americans itself is increasingly at risk, and

Americans seem to know it, if their resistance to the exchange of medical information is any indication. A *Time* magazine poll, for example, found that eighty-three percent of Americans believe that companies should be prohibited by law from selling medical information about individuals and that ninety-three percent believe that individuals should have to give their permission before such information can be made available.[4]

Promoters of the human genome project are not unmindful of the public's concern or of the potential for harm that unauthorized access to genomic information could create. At an October 1991 congressional hearing, for example, National Institutes of Health Director Bernadine Healey testified that, "Like all powerful tools, genetic information can be misused and abused. Discrimination based on genotype must be prohibited as a matter of basic civil rights."[5] At the same hearing, James Watson added "The idea that there will be a huge databank of genetic information on millions of people is repulsive."[6] Why is such a databank repulsive, and what (if anything) can be done to safeguard the genetic privacy of individuals in the genetic age?

The human genome project has the potential to alter radically our views of privacy because control of and access to the information contained in an individual's genome gives others power over the personal life of the individual. Genetic information also has its own unique privacy implications in that much genetic information about an individual will also provide information about the individual's parents, siblings, and children. The power of this information is so potentially significant that personal liberty can be protected only by stringent safeguards on access to and use of genomic information. Current policies and practices governing the privacy and confidentiality of medical information are woefully inadequate to protect personal privacy and liberty in the new genetics age. Therefore, new rules for "gene banks" (DNA sample storage facilities) are needed to help minimize the harm to individual privacy and liberty that storage of genomic information could produce.

CURRENT LAW AND PRACTICE INVOLVING MEDICAL RECORDS

Medical records provide the closest analogy to genetic samples and records. As society becomes more and more dependent on large information systems, two conflicting trends have emerged. The first trend, exemplified by state and federal Freedom of Information Acts and Sunshine Acts, is to provide the public access to information held by governmental agencies. The premise is that public knowledge of the most intimate details of how government works is likely to make government more responsive to the will of the people and to prevent official wrongdoing (such as trading arms for hostages). The second trend is exemplified by state and federal laws (such as the federal Privacy Act) designed to protect information about individual citizens from public disclosure. Details remain to be worked out in many areas. There is, however, a consensus that in all *personal* data-keeping systems, such as credit, insurance, education, taxation, criminal, and medical, individuals have or should have the right to examine and correct the information and, under most circumstances, to prevent its release without their knowledge and express authorization.

Medical records have been the last to come under public scrutiny, perhaps because medicine has a tradition of "keeping confidences." But now that sole practitioners have become an endangered species and managed care is becoming the norm, record keeping in medicine resembles other massive record-keeping systems. Accordingly, many of the rules applied to these other systems will likely be applied to medical records as well. The concept of confidentiality of medical records has been much more discussed than litigated, and only a few dozen cases have reached the appellate court level. The law in this area is still in its infancy, and resort to public policy arguments and analogy is often necessary.[7]

Almost all of the law dealing with access to medical records by people other than the patient can be categorized under the headings of confidentiality, privilege, and privacy. As commonly used, to tell someone something in confidence means that the person will not repeat the information to anyone else. *Confidentiality* presupposes that something secret will be told by someone to a second party (such as a doctor) who will not repeat it to a third party (such as an employer). Relationships such as attorney–client, priest–penitent, and doctor–patient are confidential relationships. In the doctor–patient context, confidentiality is understood as an expressed or implied agreement that the doctor will not disclose the information received from the patient to anyone not directly involved in the patient's care and treatment.

A communication is privileged if the person to whom the information is given is forbidden by law from disclosing it in a court proceeding without the consent of the person who provided it. *Privilege*, sometimes called *testimonial privilege*, is a legal rule of evidence, applying only in the judicial context. The privilege belongs to the client, not to the professional, although the hospital, physician, or data bank may have a duty to assert it on behalf of the patient. Unlike attorney–client privilege, doctor–patient privilege is not recognized as common law and therefore exists only if a state statute establishes it (and, indeed, most states have such statutes).

There are at least four senses in which the term *privacy* is generally used in a legal sense. The first three describe aspects of the constitutional right of privacy. The central one, in the liberty interests protected by the Fourteenth Amendment, is the right of privacy as autonomy that forms the basis for the opinions by the U.S. Supreme Court limiting state interference with individual *decisions* concerning birth control and abortion. This sense of privacy involves liberty because it specifically relates to an individual's ability to make important decisions that intimately affect one's personhood free from government interference. The second and third types of constitutional rights protect certain *relationships*, such as husband–wife, parent–child, and doctor–patient relationships, and certain *places*, such as the bedroom, from governmental intrusion.

In the more traditional common law sense, the right of privacy has been defined as "the right to be let alone," to be free of prying, peeping, and snooping, and as the right of someone to keep information about himself or his personality inaccessible to others. In *Privacy and Freedom*, Alan Westin defines privacy as "the claim of individuals, groups, or institutions to determine for themselves when, how, and to what extent information about them is communicated to others."[8] He goes on to argue that, as thus defined, the concept has its roots in the territorial behavior of animals, and its importance can be seen to some extent through the history of civilization. What is at stake here can be described as *informational* privacy. Many diverse acts come under the heading of privacy violations, but most involving medical records are in the informational area and can be generally described as the "publication [disclosing to one or more unauthorized person] of private matters violating ordinary decencies."[9] A court can conclude that the unauthorized disclosure of medical records (including genomic information) is an actionable invasion of privacy even without a state statute that specifically forbids it. As an Alabama court put it in a case involving disclosure of medical information by a physician to a patient's employer, "Unauthorized disclosure of intimate details of a patient's health may amount to unwarranted publication of one's private affairs with which the public has no legitimate concern, such as to cause outrage, mental suffering, shame, or humiliation to a person of ordinary sensibilities."[10]

The policy underlying the right of informational privacy is that because of the potential severe consequences to individuals, certain "private" information about them (such as their HIV status) should not be repeated without their permission. In the words of one legal commentator, "the basic attribute of an effective right of privacy is the individual's ability to control the flow of information concerning or describing him."[11] Most of the cases in the doctor–patient context alleging violation of the right to privacy have involved actions in which personal medical information has been published in a newspaper or magazine, and often the suit is against the publisher rather than the physician. In the specific case of genomic information, informational privacy, relational (family) privacy, and decision-making privacy all overlap, creating arguably unique privacy concerns.

THE CASE OF DNA PROFILING AND CRIMINAL GENE BANKS

Medical record keeping provides the major analogy for DNA sample storage, but the use of DNA in criminal records is becoming widespread as well.[12] The banking of DNA samples is useful primarily because of the technique of amplification, known as polymerase chain reaction (PCR), which permits small quantities of DNA to be multiplied into large quantities with relative ease. As this applies to criminal investigations, it means that DNA samples in trace materials (such as semen, blood, and hair) found at the scene of a crime can be compared with DNA samples from crime suspects. In addition, files of DNA profiles could be used like fingerprints to compare with profiles from a crime scene. This technology is extremely attractive to law enforcement officers and has already been used in ways that help explain why an individual might be concerned about the banking of samples of his or her DNA. DNA typing is based on the assumption that a combination of specific repetitive DNA sequences ("variable number of tandem repeats," or VNTRs) in a person is extremely unlikely to match the DNA of anyone else.[13]

A suspect can be placed at the scene of the crime in a number of ways. The most common is by an eyewitness. But eyewitnesses are notoriously unreliable, and most prosecutors prefer to have eyewitness testimony supplemented by physical evidence such as fingerprints or footprints. In violent crimes such as rape and murder, the perpetrator may leave his sperm or blood behind or carry away some of the victim's blood on his person. Using ABO blood groups, individuals can be *excluded* as suspects because their blood types do not match the sample left at the scene of the crime. By using DNA typing, however, it has been suggested that suspects can be conclusively identified as the source of blood or sperm. This type of identification has been hyped by law enforcement officials as the ultimate law enforcement tool, and its first use to help solve a murder case is graphically chronicled in Joseph Wambaugh's bestseller, *The Blooding*. A California Department of Justice official predicts that "in a few years, a crime-scene sample will tell a suspect's race, eye color, hair color and even his build." Others see DNA samples as eventually being fed into a computer that will decode them and produce "an image like the kind our police artists do now."[14]

There is general agreement that DNA profiling or fingerprinting can accurately exclude individuals from being possible suspects of specific crimes, and it should continue to be so used. However, problems have been demonstrated with some of the methods used (which have not been standardized) by the country's major private testing laboratories, and ultimately there must be national standards on laboratory procedures. In addition, issues of population genetics (used to determine the probability of a match by chance) continue to be contentious.

U.S. courts agree that DNA profiling itself is scientifically accepted, but they are currently split on the proper evidentiary standard to use in admitting DNA fingerprinting for use by the jury in a criminal trial, although the majority admit such evidence under either standard. A January 1992 decision by the U.S. Court of Appeals for the Second Circuit may set the standard.[15] The court rejected the traditional (and still majority) "*Frye* rule" in which admissability of novel scientific information is not permitted until the technique has been "sufficiently established to have gained general acceptance in the particular field in which it belongs."[16] This standard would require acceptance of population-based probability as determination as well. Instead of this "general acceptance" standard, the court adopted the newer standard of the Federal Rules of Evidence (Rule 702) which treats scientific evidence no differently than any other evidence:

> If scientific, technological, or other specialized knowledge will assist the trier of fact to understand the evidence or to determine a fact in issue, a witness qualified as an expert by knowledge, skill, expertise, training, or education, may testify thereto in the form of an opinion or otherwise.

Under this rule, according to the court, it is not for the judge to decide if what the expert says is "true," only if the expert's testimony can assist the jury in discharging "its duties of weighing the evidence, making credibility determinations, and ultimately deciding the facts." The court, noting the tendency to liberalize admissibility rules and let the jury decide, concluded that it did not think "that a jury will be so dazzled or swayed as to ignore evidence suggesting that an experiment was improperly conducted or that testing procedures have not been established." But the court decided to go much further than simply affirming the decision of the trial judge (whose procedure they concluded would also have satisfied the *Frye* rule), and rejecting the *Frye* criteria, concluded that for future cases in the Second Circuit,

> . . . a court could properly take judicial notice of the general acceptability of the general theory and the use of these specific techniques (of DNA typing). . . . The threshold of admissibility should require only a preliminary showing of reliability of the particular data to be offered, i.e., some indication of how the laboratory work was done and what analysis and assumptions underlie the probability calculations.

The court went on to acknowledge the subpopulation problem, noting that "the probability data may well vary among different segments of the population," but concluded nonetheless that "affidavits should normally suffice to provide a sufficient basis for admissibility."

Some states now condition parole on the deposit of a DNA sample with the police (in most cases for sex offenders only, but it seems inevitable that all felonies will soon be included, and then all crimes). The purpose, of course, is to be able to "locate" the perpetrator of future sex crimes among former sex offenders. It will likely be seen as reasonable at some point in the future to have the FBI store samples of everyone's DNA (just as they now have a large proportion of the population's fingerprints) to make the job of law enforcement easier. Who but criminals could object? One problem is that this approach treats everyone in the United States (whose DNA is on file) as a crime suspect, making us a "nation of suspects."[17]

The more generic gene bank problem is that once a governmental agency has a DNA sample, it can learn much more about the individual than just whether or not their DNA "matches" a sample taken from a crime scene. The agency cannot only discover the genetic makeup of an individual but also, in the future, may be able to learn about genetic predispositions—the probability of an individual developing a specific (in fact, many specific) genetically determined or genetically influenced diseases. There are currently no standards governing the use of criminal DNA banks in such ways. Accordingly, it seems most prudent at this point to limit the information that law enforcement officials can store on convicted felons and others to the actual sequences of portions of their DNA (digitalized for computer storage and use) and not to an actual DNA sample that can be used for a multitude of privacy-invading purposes unrelated to law enforcement.

DNA AS A FUTURE DIARY

DNA samples stored in gene banks contain information that is significantly more personal and private than both fingerprints and medical records. A medical record contains information about one's past; a DNA molecule contains information about one's *future* as well. A medical record can be analogized to a diary, but a DNA molecule is much more sensitive. It is in a real sense a "future diary" (although a probabilistic one), and it is written in a code that we have not yet cracked. But the code is being broken piece by piece (and this is the major goal of the human genome project) such that custodians of samples of an individual's DNA will be able to learn more and more about that individual and his or her family as the code is broken.

It seems reasonable to conclude that the mere existence of the technology to "decode" one's DNA will lead us to radically alter our view of informational privacy. In the past we have put special emphasis on information that is potentially embarrassing and sensitive (such as sexually transmitted diseases) and on information that is uniquely personal (such as a photograph of one's face). Genetic information is both potentially embarrassing and uniquely personal. It seems likely that either the existence of such decodable information will impel us to take privacy much more seriously in the genetic realm than we have in the medical and criminal realms or it will lead us to give up on maintaining personal privacy altogether. This latter response seems defeatist and unlikely. However, the success of TV programs such as *Geraldo Rivera* and *Oprah Winfrey*, which flourish on ordinary Americans discussing the intimate details of their sex lives and family problems, evidences both a voyeuristic strain in many Americans as well as an exhibitionistic trait. Is it too much to think that future guests may have their genomes "decoded" before a live studio audience or that whole families might appear for a public genomic diagnosis for Oprah? However one answers these questions, the issue of privacy and liberty revolves around *choice* in exposing personal information such as that contained in one's genome. What lessons can we learn from current information systems that might help us maintain control over our own genetic information?

RULES FOR MEDICAL INFORMATION SYSTEMS

Rules about medical information are mostly state rules, and there has been very little serious study of the problems of medical record-keeping systems since the early 1970s. At that time, when computerization of medical records was in its infancy, the U.S. Congress established the Privacy Protection Study Commission to study privacy rights and record-keeping practices generically. Its 1977 report remains the most thoughtful and authoritative statement on large record-keeping systems.[18] In regard to the medical records, the Commission found that medical records contain more information and are available to more users than ever before; that the control of health care providers over these records has been greatly diluted; that restoration of this control is not possible; that voluntary patient consent to disclosure is generally illusory; that patients' access to their records is rare; and that there are steps that can be taken to improve the quality of records, to enhance patients' awareness of their content, and to control their disclosure. Some of the commission's major recommendations are that

1. "each State enact a statute creating individual rights of access to, and correction of, medical records, and an enforceable expectation of confidentiality for medical records . . ."
2. ". . . Federal and State penal codes be amended to make it a criminal offense for any individual knowingly to request or obtain medical record information from a medical care provider under false pretenses or through deception."
3. ". . . upon request, an individual who is the subject of a medical record maintained by a medical care provider, or another responsible person designated by the individual, be allowed to have access to that medical record, including the opportunity to see and copy it." Each individual should also have the opportunity to correct or amend the record.
4. ". . . each medical care provider be required to take affirmative measures to assure that the medical records it maintains are made available only to authorized recipients and on a 'need-to-know' basis."
5. ". . . any disclosure of medical record information by a medical care provider be limited only to information necessary to accomplish the purpose for which the disclosure is made."
6. ". . . each medical care provider be required to notify an individual on whom it maintains a medical record of the disclosures that may be made of information in the record without the individual's express authorization."[19]

Of course, it is not only the storage of information that is problematic. It is the use of such information by third parties to make decisions about the future of individuals that puts an individual's privacy and liberty interests most directly at risk. The U.S. Privacy Commission was careful to specify rules for the release of data identified with a particular individual from the data bank. The Commission discovered, for example, that often when an individual applies for a job, life or health insurance, credit or financial assistance, or services from the government, the individual is asked to relinquish certain medical information. Although this is necessary in many cases, the commission found that individuals are generally asked to sign open-ended or blanket authorizations with clauses such as one requiring the recipient to "furnish any and all information on request."

It is remarkable that these rules have not been adopted. Nevertheless, if these rules are reasonable (and I think they are), they lead to some even more stringent rules for the maintenance of DNA molecules that contain an individual's probabilistic, coded future diary.

PRIVACY RULES FOR GENE BANKS

Since there are no existing privacy rules for gene banks, and since most genetic samples are now being collected and stored either by hospital-based programs or by private clinics and corporations, it seems reasonable to suggest a moratorium on such storage until reasonable rules are developed. However, because most storage (outside of law enforcement agencies) is in private hands, it seems unlikely that any agreement on a moratorium could be enforced without federal legislation. Since this itself seems unlikely, it is probably more constructive to try to get agreement on the rules that all gene banks should follow with or without legislative mandate. The following preliminary rules are suggested to protect individual privacy and liberty while permitting reasonable medical research and treatment goals to be pursued:

1. No DNA bank should be created or begin to store samples until there is
   a. public notice that the DNA bank is to be established, including the reason for the bank, and
   b. a privacy impact statement is prepared and filed with a designated public agency that is also responsible for developing and enforcing privacy guidelines for the DNA bank (ultimately, a DNA bank-licensing board should be established to license all DNA banks in the United States with uniform rules).
   c. the burden of proof should be on the DNA bank to establish that storage of DNA molecules is necessary to achieve an important medical or societal goal.
2. No collection of DNA samples destined for storage is permissible without prior written authorization of the individual that

    a. sets forth the purpose of the storage;

    b. sets forth all uses, including any and all commercial uses, that will be permitted of the DNA sample;

    c. guarantees the individual (i) continued access to the sample and all records about the sample and (ii) the absolute right to order the identifiable sample destroyed at any time; and

    d. guarantees the destruction of the sample or its return to the individual should the DNA bank significantly change its identity or cease operation.

3. DNA samples can only be used for the purposes for which they are collected. Specifically, as protection against unwanted and unforeseeable uses, there may be

    a. no waivers or "boilerplate" statements that permit other uses;

    b. no access to the DNA information by any third party without written notification to the individual, whose sample is being used;

    c. no access by third parties to any personally identifiable information; and

    d. strict security measures, including criminal penalties for misuse or unauthorized use of DNA information.

4. Mechanisms must be developed to notify and counsel those whose DNA samples are in storage when new information that can have a significant health impact on the individual is obtainable from their stored DNA sample.[20]

Most of these proposed rules are self-explanatory. It may seem premature to develop rules or guidelines for DNA banks, but the long history of medical record keeping, and the short history of DNA fingerprinting demonstrates that standards *are* necessary. Some questions these proposals have raised merit comment. First, where is the "designated public agency" responsible for developing and enforcing privacy guidelines? The response—that there currently is no such agency—is not satisfactory. There should be one, and ideally it should be a federal agency because few, if any, DNA banks will operate solely within the confines of any one state. This agency should be as independent as possible from the funding agencies (such as the National

Institute of Health) and could be an independent agency such as the Nuclear Regulatory Commission.

The requirements for "informed storage" are not remarkable and are analogous to both medical records storage and embryo storage. Embryos are even more important than DNA samples since they have the potential to become children. Typical storage contracts currently require the couple to agree to such things as disposition of the embryos upon the separation, divorce, or death of one or both of the couple, as well as limiting the terms of the storage and providing for other contingencies. Even more elaborate storage agreements are used when an individual wants his or her entire body frozen and stored for possible "treatment" at some distant time in the future. The point is not that we should treat DNA samples like embryos or bodies but that detailed storage contracts and consent forms are not a novel idea and can be implemented.

The use restrictions are in relatively standard privacy protection language, although many researchers and commercial enterprises might object to keeping track of current addresses and to the requirement forbidding all third-party access to identifiable information. In the research context, the practice has been to appeal to the Institutional Review Board (IRB) for such uses, but this is very unsatisfactory. The IRB does not approve the new use when the sample is collected, and the individual cannot have given his or her consent (at which time it is usually just as easy to get a new sample) *unless* the type of research is agreed to at the time the sample is collected. Obviously, this agreement cannot be generic (e.g., "all genetic research"), but it *could* include specific types of research not currently envisioned (e.g., "all attempts to locate CF [cystic fibrosis] genes")

The final rule is the one that requires the most work to make operational. Since most new genetic tests often appear first in the nation's newspapers, notification may be less important than counseling options.[21] Each DNA bank could also have a newsletter that it routinely sends to all depositors, and any new genetic tests could be described therein. It seems unlikely that the "duty to protect" the depositor's family members would ever arise at a storage facility, although research facilities may discover a genetic condition that has serious implications for family members. If this is a possibility, the facility's policy on such disclosure should be made clear at the time of deposit so that the individual who disagrees with it can keep his or her DNA sample out of that bank.

As should be evident from this discussion, these are preliminary proposals that require additional discussion, debate, and refinement. There certainly is room and need for this discussion. The issues at stake, however, are privacy and liberty, and compromises in the security of the data contained in the DNA molecule will ultimately compromise the privacy and liberty of the individuals whose DNA are stored in DNA banks. Scientists, physicians, and the public should take a strong stand in favor of privacy.

In this regard, James Watson's comments on the "repulsive" nature of huge databanks are on target. It is, of course, not the gene banks per se that are repulsive but the seemingly inevitable misuse of the data stored in them to the detriment of individual citizens. For example, we may tolerate a consulting physician discussing Magic Johnson's HIV status in the *New York Times* without sanctioning that same physician running a DNA profile on Johnson to discover and then disclose any genetic conditions or predispositions he might carry. Likewise, some commentators have found it acceptable for Martin Orne to discuss his therapy sessions with Anne Sexton's biographer. Nonetheless, even these commentators would likely want to prohibit current biographers of Sexton from examining her DNA to discover what genetically determined conditions she may have suffered from. This could be out of a concern either for the future privacy of all of us or for the current privacy of Anne Sexton's children, whose privacy would also be invaded by disclosing her DNA profile. And even in the case of Abraham Lincoln, whose relatives are all long deceased, a greater justification than simple curiosity should be required for historians to be given access to his DNA.

Most of us, of course, will not be the subject of front page news stories, biographers, or historians. It will be the police, our insurance company, our employers, and our families that are most likely to seek the information encoded in our DNA. If we are to stand any reasonable chance of keeping this information confidential, we will need early agreement on some basic rules for gene banks. Without such agreement, the two unattractive alternatives would seem to be abandoning current notions of privacy and confidentiality or outlawing DNA banks altogether.

Although written in the pregenomic era and with no thought of gene banks in mind, some lines of Anne Sexton's poetry provide a fitting conclusion (and a hopeful note) for this chapter:

Each cell has a life.
There is enough here to please a nation.
It is enough that the populace own these goods.
Any person, any commonwealth would say of it,
"It is good this year that we may plant again
and think forward to a harvest.
A blight had been forecast and has been cast out."[22]

NOTES

An earlier version of this paper was presented at a workshop on "The Impact of Molecular Genetics on Society," held at the Banbury Center, Cold Springs Harbor, New York, 5–8 Nov. 1990. I would also like to acknowledge the comments on the proposed "rules" by the participants at a AAAS/ABA Conference on Ethical and Legal Aspects of Large Pedigree Genetic Research, Wild Dunes, Charleston, South Carolina, 13–15 March 1992, which were of great assistance in completing this paper.

1. Diane Wood Middlebrook, *Anne Sexton: A Biography* (Boston: Houghton Mifflin, 1991). See also "Confidentiality in Psychotherapy—The Case of Anne Sexton," *New England Journal of Medicine* 325 (1991): 1450–1451.

2. L. K. Altman, "Johnson Will Get Drug Treatment To Fight Virus," *New York Times*, 9 November 1991, p. 33.

3. Ibid.

4. R. Lacayo, "Nowhere to Hide," *Time*, 11 November 1991, 34–40. And see M. W. Millerm, "Patients' Records are Treasure Trove for Budding Industry," *Wall Street Journal*, 27 February 1992, p. 1.

5. C. Anderson, "Evolution of a Gadfly," *Nature* 353 (1991): 686–687.

6. Ibid.

7. G. J. Annas, *The Rights of Patients* (Carbondale, IL: Southern Illinois Univ. Press, 1989), 175–195.

8. Allan Westin, *Privacy and Freedom* (New York: Atheneum, 1967), 7.

9. Ibid.

10. *Horne v. Patton*, 291 Ala. 701, 287 So. 2d 824 (1973).

11. Miller, "Personal privacy in the computer age," 67 *Mich. L. Rev.* 1091, 1107 (1968).

12. Portions of this section were adapted from G. J. Annas, "DNA Fingerprinting in the Twilight Zone," *Hastings Center Report* 20 (1990): 35–37.

13. The standard method of DNA fingerprinting uses the same restriction fragment length polymorphism (RFLP) analysis used in genetic testing and screening. Restriction enzymes recognize and cut specific nucleotide sequences in DNA molecules. Since the nucleotide sequences in the human

genome vary widely from person to person, the restriction sites will also vary and therefore the length and content of the fragments. RFLP analysis rests on the finding that two samples of DNA from the same individual will produce the same DNA fragments, whereas samples from different individuals (other than identical twins) will produce different fragments from the same site. See G. J. Annas, "Setting Standards for the Use of DNA-Typing Results in the Courtroom—The State of the Art," *New England Journal of Medicine* 326 (1992):1641.

14. Quoted in Annas, "DNA Fingerprinting," 36.

15. *U.S. v. Jakobetz,* 955 F.2d 786 (2d Cir. 1992); *State v. Two Bulls,* 918 F. 2d 56 (8th Cir. 1990).

16. *Frye v. U.S.,* 293 F. 1013 (D.C. Cir. 1923).

17. L. H. Glantz, "A Nation of Suspects: Drug Testing and the Fourth Amendment," *American Journal of Public Health* 79 (1989): 1427–1431. See also P. Aldhous, "Challenge to British Forensic Database," *Nature* 355 (1992): 191.

18. Privacy Protection Study Commission, *Personal Privacy in an Information Society* (Washington D.C.: U.S. Government Printing Office, 1977).

19. The recommendations quoted and summarized here are among the fourteen made on pages 292–317 in *Personal Privacy in an Information Society.*

20. George J. Annas and Sherman Elias, eds., *Gene Mapping: Using Law and Ethics as Guides* (New York: Oxford University Press, 1992), 9–10; George J. Annas, "Privacy Rules for DNA Databases Protecting Coded 'Future Diaries,' " *Journal of the American Medical Association* 270 (1993): 2346–2350.

21. See, e.g., Gina Kolata, "Cancer-Causing Gene Found; with a Clue to How it Works," *New York Times,* 6 May 1993, p. A1.

22. From Anne Sexton, "In Celebration of My Uterus," in *Love Poems* (Boston: Houghton Mifflin, 1967).

6

USE OF GENETIC INFORMATION BY PRIVATE INSURERS

Robert J. Pokorski

Because a great deal of the present concern regarding future use of genetic information by insurers stems from a lack of knowledge of the basic tenets of private, voluntary insurance, I would like to overview briefly some of the fundamental principles of private insurance before directly addressing issues associated with advances in genetic technology. It will be the goal of this essay to describe not only those principles but to argue that genetic information must be made available to insurers as a matter of equity.

PRINCIPLES OF INSURANCE

Insurance is intended to provide financial protection against unexpected or untimely events. In particular, life and health insurance are purchased not in anticipation of imminent death or illness—although it is understood that death is inevitable and serious illness is fairly common. Rather, life insurance is obtained to protect dependents or business associates from the financial disadvantages that can occur in the event of unexpected death, and health insurance is meant to provide protection in the event of a significant financial loss associated with an unanticipated illness.

How does private insurance work? Basically, policyholders pay a relatively small, affordable amount into a common "pool," and the benefits of the pool are distributed to the unfortunate few who die (life insurance), become disabled (disability insurance), or develop illness (health insurance). In this way, the financial loss attendant to these events can be mitigated even through the events themselves cannot be prevented.

But not all people are alike. The likelihood of occurrence and magnitude of loss varies across those differences. Some people apply for large amounts of insurance and others for small amounts. Some are young and others elderly. Occupations and avocations modify the likelihood of unexpected death or illness, as do health-enhancing activities such as exercise, proper diet, and not smoking. And some applicants are already in poor health or at known significant risk of developing poor health in the future. These different factors are evaluated by the insurance company through a process known as "risk selection and classification." The more common term for this process is "underwriting." Through underwriting, the insurance company determines the appropriate contribution to the risk pool by an individual policyholder.

The fundamental goal of the underwriting process is equity: policyholders with the same or similar expected risk of loss are charged the same. The higher the risk, the higher the premium. The lower the risk, the lower the premium. Note the distinction between equity and equality. With *equity*, premiums vary by risk; with *equality*, everyone—young or old, healthy or ill, and with or without associated factors that significantly increase the likelihood of making an early claim—would pay the same price.

During the underwriting process, risk classifications are created that recognize the many differences that exist among individuals in order to place applicants into groups with comparable expectations of longevity and health. Although the risk presented by any single individual cannot be determined with absolute precision, if people are assigned to groups with reasonable accuracy and the total number of insured people is large, then the estimate of the risk of the entire group of insured people is likely to be accurate.

Traditionally, characteristics important for risk classification have included factors such as age, gender, health history, physical condition, occupation, the use of alcohol and tobacco, family history, and serum cholesterol. These factors serve to identify individuals that have a greater or lesser likelihood of premature death or illness in the future. Because of this process, costs are held down for the great majority of insurance applicants since premiums more closely match the risks taken on by the insurance company.

How are rates determined that reflect the principle of equity? Under state laws and in the opinion of most observers, rates are considered equitable when they allow the insurer to earn enough income to pay claims and expenses and generate a reasonable margin for the risks they accept. In other words,

> rates should be *adequate* but not excessive and should *discriminate* fairly between insureds. They should be adequate in order to provide insurers with sufficient income. They should not be excessive, for excessive rates impose undue burden on insureds. And they should discriminate fairly so that each insured will pay in accordance with the quality of his life.[1]

The previous statement reflects the rate-setting philosophy of a private insurance company—not *equal* but *equitable* treatment of all. It recognizes differences among classes of insured persons, with products priced at a level that will result in a payment by each insured of an amount that is fair. Such fairness is accomplished by equating the anticipated cost to the company and the amount of the premium.

The vocabulary of insurance can be confusing. In the context of private insurance, *discrimination* is not necessarily bad and *equality* good. For example, in accordance with the insurance philosophy just set out, it would not be equitable to collect the same annual premium for the same life coverage from a sixty-year-old man in poor health as collected from a twenty-year-old woman in good health. To charge an *equal* premium would be inequitable. An insurer may—and must—discriminate to achieve equity, insofar as the discrimination remains fair. In fact, the statutes, regulations, and case laws that regulate the insurance industry compel discrimination; what they forbid is *unfair* discrimination.

Adverse selection, also known as antiselection, is a consideration that is of great importance to insurers. *Adverse selection* is a well-known phenomenon. It occurs when people with a greater likelihood of loss than what they are charged for continue insurance coverage to a greater extent than other people. It occurs when applicants withhold significant information from the insurer and/or choose amounts and types of insurance that are most beneficial to themselves. For example, someone with a history of heart disease is more likely to apply for insurance and/or apply for a greater amount of insurance coverage than he would have otherwise done because he knows that he is likely to experience a claim in the foreseeable future. If he fails to mention this important information on his insurance application and the insurer does not otherwise become aware of it, the premium charged by the insurer will be insufficient to cover the risk involved. This premium deficit would be made up by the others in the pool who have paid their fair share. Adverse selection also occurs if the insurer is not permitted to obtain or use information that is pertinent to the risk being considered. In this example, the premiums charged would be insufficient to cover the risk involved if the insurer was not permitted to ask the proposed insured and his attending physician about the nature and severity of the heart disease or if this information could not be used in setting premium cost after it had been obtained.

What would happen if the insurance company were unaware of important, unfavorable information that was known to the applicant? In these instances, serious errors in risk classification would occur. Certain individuals would receive their insurance at unreasonably low cost. More claims would be filed than were expected, and if a significant number of these risk classification errors were made, the financial status of the entire insurance pool would be adversely affected.

But could premiums simply be increased across the board to cover the payment of these unanticipated benefits? Where permitted, an insurer could increase premiums to reflect these revised claim expectations. But this would encourage potential insurance applicants who are at lower risk to either buy from a different seller or exit the insurance market altogether. And for the individuals who had knowledge of their unfavorable risk status—individuals who had adversely selected against the insurance pool—further escalation of premiums would become necessary. More potential applicants would then decide not to apply for insurance.

Eventually, a point is reached in this upward spiral where the desired coverage becomes unavailable on any reasonable premium basis or the insurer becomes financially unsound. This "assessment spiral" is not merely a theoretical possibility. It actually occurred in some companies during the 1880s and 1890s because of poor risk classification practices. A more recent example of the effects of failing to classify risks properly is provided by the recent failure of a moderate-sized casualty insurer located in Chicago.[2] The company originally specialized in individual disability income policies. In the early 1970s, new management took over the company and decided to use its casualty authority to write auto insurance. They believed that people living in some of Chicago's neighborhoods were being charged auto premiums that were too high. Based on this belief, management ignored the actuarial statistics and evidence and wrote auto insurance for drivers in these neighborhoods at rates that would have been correct for a population with far fewer auto accidents. As a result, the company failed and everyone involved was hurt financially. All the company's lines of business were affected, including its disability income line. Many disabled individuals who had long depended on income payments lost those benefits.

The current risk classification system permits private insurers throughout the world to respond fairly to valid cost and experience-related differences among persons. To help guide actuaries in developing this system, the actuarial profession through the Actuarial Standards Board has adopted a risk classification standard of practice. This standard enumerates three basic requirements for an appropriate risk classification system. First, risk classification must be fair. Second, it must permit economic incentives to operate and thus encourage widespread availability of coverage in the marketplace. Finally, risk classification must do its part to keep the insurer solvent. To achieve these ends, a sound classification system should be based on at least four principles:

1. Risk classifications should reflect cost and experience differences. For example, employers of coal miners would pay more for their unemployment insurance than employers of computer technicians because coal miners historically have much higher rates of unemployment.
2. The system should be applied objectively and consistently. By this principle, for example, males of the same age with similar health histories would be charged similar rates for life insurance.
3. The system should be practical, cost effective, and responsive to change. This means that there would be limits on how much effort and money could be spent to classify a given risk and that risk

classification systems must be dynamic. For instance, when polio was eliminated as a public health hazard, the system changed to reflect that development.

4. Adverse selection should be minimized. As noted earlier, sound risk classification systems limit the ability of an applicant to take an unfair financial advantage at the expense of the insurance company or other policyholders already insured by the company.

PRIVATE AND PUBLIC INSURANCE

Many people have come to expect that private life insurance and, to a greater extent, private health insurance, is an entitlement, that is, that all citizens have a right to expect that affordable insurance protection will be made available to them regardless of age or health. This expectation is based to a considerable degree on misconceptions regarding the nature of private versus public insurance programs. A brief discussion of these two different types of insurance will help clarify their relationships.

Private (Voluntary) Insurance   Participation in a private commercial insurance plan is typically voluntary. An individual chooses whether or not to belong and determines how much insurance protection he or she would like to purchase. Since all of the funds used to pay future claims against the insurance pool are derived either directly or indirectly from premium payments, risk classification is essential to ensure that the premium charged is proportionate to the risk assumed. The potential for adverse selection is very real and an important concern of the insurer. Finally, private insurance companies are businesses that are accountable to their policyholders and stockholders. They must generate a profit for those who have invested in the company. If insufficient premiums are collected, a private insurance company, like any other business in which liabilities exceed assets, will cease to exist.

Public (Involuntary) Insurance   American society has used private means to fulfill certain general social welfare needs such as payment for health care. But private health insurance has never been a completely adequate or universal method of providing access to the health care system, nor has it been a perfect mechanism for covering all diseases. The poor, disabled, aged, or seriously ill cannot always be covered by private means. For this reason, society has supplemented private insurance with publicly supported programs such as Social Security, Medicaid, and Medicare.

Participation in a public insurance plan is not typically voluntary. One does not choose whether or not to belong nor does one determine the extent of insurance protection. Rather, participation is mandatory, and benefit amounts or entitlements are determined by the law establishing the program. Since everyone—good risks, poor risks, even those suffering from a severe or terminal illness—is automatically insured and there are no options regarding the amount of benefits that will be paid, adverse selection is not a concern. Premiums are charged in the form of income and social security taxes, or so-called insurance premiums, but they are not and need not be proportionate to the risk assumed. Risk selection is not required and no profit motive exists.

The foregoing points comparing private and public insurance are summarized in Table 6.1.

Even given these fundamental differences between private commercial insurance and public insurance, could legislators or regulators simply mandate that private insurers provide coverage—at rates appropriate for lower risks—to those individuals who have learned from their physicians or insurer that a genetic test has identified a higher likelihood of premature death or illness? Or, in an action having the same consequences, could insurers be prohibited from asking applicants and their physicians for the results of prior genetic tests or order their own tests?

There seems little chance that this would work in a private voluntary insurance industry. This mandated subsidization of unfavorable risks by good risks would be tantamount to an indirect governmental tax levied solely against insurance policyholders and stockholders. The impact of such an action may not appear significant at the outset, but its cumulative effects would be dramatic. Under such a scenario, many potential policyholders—primarily favorable risks who would be asked to subsidize the higher, underpriced risks

Table 6.1 Comparisons Between Private and Public Insurers

	Private (Voluntary) Insurance)	*Public (Involuntary) Insurance*
Examples	Private, commercial insurers	Medicare, Medicaid, Social Security
Participation	Voluntary	Mandatory
Amount of insurance	Optional	Controlled
Risk classification	Essential	Unnecessary
Potential for adverse selection	Yes	Unnecessary
Profit required	Yes	No

and people with other health impairments such as cancer and heart disease who pay a premium commensurate with their increased risk— would realize that they are being overcharged or treated unfairly and would choose not to buy insurance because coverage has now become unaffordable for them. Why? After all, the premium increase would be relatively small. Although such a plan for mandated benefits probably would not result in significantly higher costs at first, premiums would gradually and progressively rise as more and more favorable risks decide not to purchase insurance. As the relatively large base of good (standard) risks was progressively eroded, it would become increasingly difficult to subsidize the poorer risks and premiums would increase again. The situation would worsen even more as some companies would decide to stop writing this type of insurance coverage altogether because a profit could no longer be expected.

Such a legislative or regulatory mandate would force insurers to provide coverage for a large (because of the effects of adverse selection) group of people at a price that would be insufficient to cover the claims that would occur. These additional costs would be passed directly to other policyholders with a subsequent decrease in insurance affordability and availability.

INDIVIDUAL AND GROUP INSURANCE

There is yet another issue worth discussing prior to specific mention of the use of genetic test results, and that is the matter of insurance provided through employers. A brief overview of the differences between individual and group insurance is necessary in order to assess the impact of genetic testing and the arguments regarding access to test results.

For individual life, disability, and health insurance, an applicant applies for whatever amount of insurance coverage that he or she feels is needed (within broad guidelines established by the insurance company). An application form is completed, medical questions are asked, tests may be ordered, and a physician's statement may be requested. The premium charged is based on factors such as age, gender, health history, general physical condition, and occupation.

Group life and health insurance, by contrast, is generally divided into two categories: medium- to large-sized groups containing ten to twenty-five or more employees, and small groups with fewer people. Under a medium- to large-sized group life and health insurance plan, an employer buys a single policy for his or her employees. All employees can elect to receive coverage if they so choose. Benefit amounts are fixed by formula and individuals are normally not subjected to the underwriting process previously described, with the possible exceptions of those who choose not to participate in the program when they first become eligible and those who withdraw from the plan and later request reinstatement. Rather, the entire group is underwritten according to factors such as the number of employees, age and gender distribution, area of the country, and prior health care costs for the entire group. Once a rate is established, it is typically adjusted ("experience rated") on a yearly basis, depending on claims experience. If claims exceed expectations, rates increase. Or rates decrease if claims are less than expected. With such a large group, it is expected that some workers will be poor insurance risks. But the majority who are good risks tend to offset these few, thus allowing the insurer to offer coverage to the entire group at an affordable rate. Typically, payment by the employer of part of the cost provides adequate incentive for the good risks to join the insured group.

Small group life and health insurance is different. Since these groups do not have the benefit of a large number of employees among whom the health risks can be shared, claims experience is strongly dependent on the health of the small number of individuals within the group. For example, if one individual in the group was already ill or at significant risk of becoming ill in the near future, and the insurer was not aware of this information, then the claims submitted by this one individual could far exceed the claims expected from the entire group. To guard against this possibility, in the absence of underwriting, the insurer would have to increase the premium rates for all small groups. The increased premium rates would induce groups with more good risks not to buy coverage. An assessment spiral much like that described earlier for individual insurance would develop. And if such a practice occurred with any regularity, the cost of insurance to small groups would soon become unaffordable. For this reason, the underwriting of small groups shares many similarities with that of individual insurance, that is, the need for application forms, medical questions, and sometimes tests and physician reports. The principle differences between individual and group insurance are summarized in Table 6.2. The column headed "Group" refers to medium- to large-sized group plans.

Approximately ninety percent of commercial group health insurance—and perhaps a similar percentage of group life insurance—is sold to medium- to large-sized groups. The employees within these groups are eligible for insurance coverage as a benefit of their employment. There is no individual underwriting or testing of those who sign up for the program when the group plan goes into effect or when new employees begin work. For this reason, the overall impact of genetic advances on group insurance can be expected to be minimal. For small groups, the ramifications are less certain. The effects may be more like those expected for individual life and health insurance. In this regard, it is worth considering the nature of genetic disorders to see the significance of testing for these forms of insurance.

TYPES OF GENETIC DISORDERS

Genetic disorders can be divided into two broad groups: (1) disorders that follow a genetic predisposition and (2) diseases that are independent of environment.

Disorders with a genetic predisposition (or a genetic component) are those in which the presence of a gene confers an increased tendency to develop a certain disorder. The disorder may or may not develop depending on a variety of associated personal and environ-

Table 6.2 Comparisons Between Individual and Group Insurance

	Individual	*Group*
Adverse selection	Optional at discretion of an individual	Generally guaranteed as a benefit of employment; high participation is common
Amount of insurance	Optional	Controlled
Individual risk classification	Essential	Generally not done
Potential for adverse selection	Significant	Minimal

mental factors such as geographic location, diet, exposure to harmful chemicals or toxins, exercise habits, obesity, tobacco use, heavy alcohol ingestion, and so on. A genetic predisposition is often a factor in the development of common impairments such as cancer, coronary heart disease, hypertension, diabetes mellitus, and epilepsy. Together these disorders are responsible for much of the morbidity and mortality that is experienced in insurance claims.

Genetic disorders that are independent of environment involve a determining force so overwhelming that the disorder is expressed in a predictable manner without environmental interaction. For example, an individual who inherits the gene for Huntington's disease or for Duchenne muscular dystrophy will eventually develop the disorder regardless of other socioeconomic factors or preventive health measures. Individual genetic diseases are rare compared to disorders with a genetic predisposition, but collectively they are also an important cause of morbidity and mortality.

Given the genomic profiling that the human genome project is expected to make possible, physicians will probably begin to use new diagnostic tests that will enable identification of genetic diseases and predispositions to such disorder. Some of this information may be important to private insurers. Why? If this information were unavailable at the time of underwriting, then applicants who knew they were likely to experience early death or illness could buy large amounts of insurance coverage at prices that failed to reflect this increased risk. In the aggregate, this could involve disproportionately large numbers of applicants and/or very significant amounts of insurance. The ensuing claims would markedly exceed projected losses, and everyone within the insurance pool would suffer the disadvantage.

Consider the following scenario. Suppose a man who applies for an individual life or noncancelable disability insurance policy has had a genetic test performed in the past by his physician, the results are unfavorable, that is, the test suggests a significant likelihood of premature death or disability, and the insurance company does not learn about this result. If no other unfavorable risk factors are known in this case, the policy is issued on a standard class basis.

What has happened? Essentially, the principle of equity has been violated. This applicant with an above average risk for claims has obtained insurance at standard rates. This situation is analogous to that of an older person who misrepresents her true age and obtains insurance at the rates of a much younger person. It is important to note that the man in our example has not suddenly become a standard insurance risk because he was issued standard insurance. Rather, he is a substandard risk who has nonetheless obtained insurance at standard rates because of a failure of the underwriting process. Although the applicant would be pleased with this arrangement, the other policyholders would be equally unhappy with this sequence of events. True, he currently seems in good health, but his unfavorable genetic test clearly identified a significantly increased risk. And since his insurance coverage cannot be canceled once it has been purchased and neither can the premium be increased relative to other policies issued to individuals with similar coverage, it is likely that he will be paid benefits from the pool that are disproportionate to the premiums he paid.

This example is just one of the many that can be expected in the way of the genome project. Indeed, genetic advances are forcing society to confront unexpected medical, ethical, and social dilemmas. In light of the foregoing discussion about the nature and practices of insurance in the United States, four concerns of particular interest with respect to insurers' use of genomic profiling are considered next.

HOW WILL GENETIC INFORMATION
BE USED BY INSURERS?

It can be expected that genetic descriptions of individuals will be used much like other data that are developed during the underwriting process. Current tests that can be used in that process include electrocardiograms, liver and renal function tests, tests for blood sugar and cholesterol values, lung function tests, and urinalysis. Related data of interest include age, past medical history, geographic location, occupation, avocation, smoking habits, history of drug abuse or heavy alcohol ingestion, hypertension, family history, exercise, weight, and data from a physical examination. All of these factors are evaluated, and their potential impact on longevity and health is estimated. The great majority of applicants will be found to present an average risk. Some will be at lower risk, and the risk will be higher for a small number of applicants.

Genetic information would be one additional factor that is evaluated during underwriting. For example, suppose a genetic test could identify those at lower or higher risk of coronary heart disease. Favorable genetic information would tend to offset unfavorable parameters such as a high cholesterol level or hypertension. And the converse would be true for those with less favorable genetic traits.

WILL GENETIC INFORMATION AFFECT THE AVAILABILITY
OF INSURANCE COVERAGE?

It is likely that use of genetic information will not significantly affect the availability and affordability of private insurance coverage. As noted earlier, a great deal of the life and health insurance in the United States is provided on a group basis by employers. In these instances, individual underwriting is not done. Genetic information, whether favorable or unfavorable to an individual, is not likely by itself to alter these patterns of insurance provision.

In regard to individual insurance, genetic information may improve an insurer's ability to select risks in some cases, but I doubt that it will significantly affect the number of people who obtain insurance overall. As with other data developed during the underwriting process, genetic information might identify more or fewer favorable risk factors. This information, however, would be interpreted in the context of all other available data, especially since genetic diagnoses would not supplant already existing diagnostic tests and because genetic diagnoses do not always rule out insurability. Many genetic diseases, such as Down's syndrome, cystic fibrosis, and sickle cell anemia, strike very early in life and can be detected by means other than genetic tests. Having genetic tests available might not result in many additional people being identified as being at risk for these diseases. Other genetic diseases develop only late in life, with the result that young people who are predisposed to them may still have a long life expectancy. And if they have passed the age at which the disorder usually develops, their life expectancy might be normal.

There are some genetic disorders, such as Huntington's disease, for which additional genetic information might increase an individual's chance of obtaining insurance. For instance, if one parent had Huntington's disease, fifty percent of the children are at risk for the same condition. These individuals are very high mortality risks and may not be able to buy individual life coverage. Even in this case, however, a favorable genetic test result would identify those who are at virtually no risk, and insurance could be offered to them at standard rates. Many genetic predispositions involve only an increased likelihood of developing a disease, such as lung cancer, which is very uncommon in the average person. In many cases, this may not itself represent a very large increase in life insurance risk, especially if the disease is one which, like heart disease and many forms of cancer, tends to strike at relatively advanced ages.

Moreover, since genetic information may help insurers evaluate risks more precisely, there may be *fewer* rejections—not more—in the future than there are now. One reason for the rejections that occasionally occur now (in about three percent of individual life insurance applications) is that, in high risk cases, it is often impossible on the basis of present knowledge to make a close estimate of the level of risk. Presumably, an applicant would not accept a policy bearing a very high premium charge unless he or she had reason to believe that, high though the premium might be, the insurer had nevertheless underestimated the risk. The insurer, therefore, may reject such applicants rather than make an offer on a losing proposition. With greater precision in risk evaluation, the insurer would have less fear of accepting certain risks.

It is worth noting, finally, that private insurers—and not the government or other social agencies—have been responsible for initiating efforts to provide insurance coverage for people with illnesses that had been previously considered uninsurable. For example, at the turn of the century, diabetes mellitus was often fatal soon after its onset. After insulin was discovered, insurers were able to study the medical literature to determine the many different patterns of longevity and health among those with diabetes. Because they could analyze this data, classify the risks appropriately, and charge a price commensurate with the risk, insurers began to insure diabetics. The same can be said about coronary heart disease, hypertension, and many cancers.

WILL CONFIDENTIALITY OF GENETIC INFORMATION BE MAINTAINED?

Insurers have used genetic information in the underwriting process for a long time. Applications for insurance policies frequently seek information relative to family medical history, cholesterol, hypertension, coronary heart disease, cancer, diabetes, and many other impairments with a genetic component. Applicants' medical records, obtained in connection with some applications for coverage, may also reveal information relative to genetic impairments. Historically, insurers have used this information responsibly, protecting its confidentiality and relying upon it to make fair underwriting decisions. The lack of complaints about any breaches of confidentiality bear witness to this fact. Given this fine track record, I think the insurance-buying public can anticipate that any genetic information seen by insurers will be treated with the utmost confidentiality.

IS USE OF GENETIC INFORMATION BY INSURERS DISCRIMINATORY?

Much of the concern about use of genetic information by insurers stems from the word *discrimination*. In today's world, this word often carries very negative connotations, but it is a word with several means, some negative, some positive.

As noted earlier, private insurance by its very nature is recognized as being discriminatory in that individuals who represent a higher risk are routinely charged a higher premium rate. Risk selection is properly performed and there is "fair" discrimination when the applicant's expected future mortality and morbidity have been properly estimated and reflected in the premium rate. "Unfair" discrimination, in contrast, is not and should not be permitted. Unfairness in the insurance context occurs when there is no sound actuarial justification for the manner in which risks are classified.

Comments about discrimination with respect to insurers' use of genetic information highlight the mistaken impression that identifying differences in risk is somehow bad or unfair. They also indirectly express the belief that it is acceptable to "discriminate" against those with health impairments such as cancer or coronary heart disease by charging an extra premium even though these disorders are no more one's fault than are genetic impairments. Distinguishing risks is precisely what insurance companies must and, in fact, are expected to do. It is because insurers are able to identify these differences that insurance coverage can be offered to so many people at affordable rates.

Who suffers if an insurer does not charge an appropriate premium solely because the applicant's impairment has a genetic basis? The answer is healthy individuals paying standard insurance rates, policyholders who are making additional premium payments because of some nongenetic health problem, and in cases involving genetic data, the great majority of applicants whose genetic information is favorable. All of these people would be forced to pay higher rates so that those at greater risk could pay less than is required by an equitable estimate of their own risks. The attractiveness of private insurance for everyone, healthy and impaired, begins to decrease under such a schema.

Insurers try to charge premiums commensurate with risk. Applicants with a greater likelihood of experiencing an early claim are asked to pay more into the insurance pool since their risk is greater. It is this probability that is important, not whether a disease has a genetic basis or whether it can be controlled. For example, an individual with coronary heart disease or a recent history of cancer has an increased risk of death and illness. An insurer does not ask if it is or is not the individual's fault. Likewise, someone with a similar probability of early death or poor health due to a genetic disorder would be charged a similar amount. Again, fault or lack of control over the condition is not an issue.

Within the context of discrimination, the point is sometimes raised that society has prohibited the insurer's use of certain factors over which a person has no control, notably race, gender, and religion, even though these are characteristics that would be useful to consider when trying to classify risks. Given this kind of moral precedent, so the argument goes, society should also prohibit use of genetic information in classifying risks. This is a serious issue and deserves a response.

First, it is true that insurers are legally prohibited from basing underwriting decisions on race. It is also worth emphasizing that insurers are very supportive of this legislation. The reason is this: race by itself is not a risk factor in determining an individual's expectations for health and longevity. Differences in morbidity and mortality among races are explained by the presence of health impairments. Laws prohibiting use of race during the underwriting process are in essence a confirmation of the principle of equity. They state that risks that are equal—that is, the intrinsically equal morbidity and mortality among races—must be treated the same. Note that they do not require that insurers treat different risks the same, as would be the case if such a philosophy were applied to those at greater risk of death or illness because of cancer, heart disease, or a genetic impairment.

Regarding gender, epidemiological experts have concluded that there are intrinsic gender-related differences in morbidity and mortality risks. These gender-related differences are recognized in the vast majority of jurisdictions. As of July 1991, for example, there were no federal laws or regulations mandating unisex pricing for life or health insurance products. And only one state—Montana—has enacted unisex legislation that affects life and health insurance. This bill was passed in 1983, and there have been repeated attempts to repeal it since that time.

I am unaware if insurers ever used religion to classify risks. The members of some religious groups such as Mormons and Seventh-Day Adventists have high average longevity, certainly attributable in part to a principled avoidance of alcohol and tobacco use. Legislation requiring insurers to treat all religious backgrounds equally would presumably have the unintended effect of a prohibition of offering *lower cost* coverage on this basis.

CONCLUSIONS

Diagnostic and therapeutic advances in the practice of medicine are both inevitable and desirable. The genetic testing one may expect in the wake of the human genome project offers exactly such advances. Genetic testing will be thrust on a society that has had little experience in dealing with many of the complex ethical, medical, and social issues that will ensue. Many facets of society—including the private insurance industry—will need to study the potential impact of this new technology and adapt to it. At this time, insurers are no more able to answer the difficult questions concerning future use of genetic testing than is any other facet of society. In fact, most of the questions themselves are still unknown. We will continue to study the issues and await further developments. This can be the only reasonable course of action until significant technological advances are made and the nature and use of genetic testing becomes more apparent.

What insurers fear most in the future is that people will learn of important, personal genetic information outside the context of insurance and then successfully use this medical knowledge to gain an undue advantage in the application process. This is unfair both to insurers and other applicants and policyholders who must pay higher premiums so that coverage can be issued to those who fail to disclose this information. Americans choose the type of insurance system they want. If they choose a private insurance system, it must be one that makes sound decisions about which risks it will insure. A system that does not classify risks will at some point cease to be an "insurance" system. Whatever entitlement program remains will be very expensive because it will allow unrestricted access to coverage by those with very serious diseases, some of which are genetic in nature.

There are those who would suggest that genetic information not be shared with insurers, this in spite of the likelihood that this information will be favorable in the great majority of cases. As noted in a recent editorial dealing with ethics and the human genome, "A rule that insurance companies should not seek genetic information about potential policyholders would probably be unenforceable, would be unjust to those free from defect, and would probably be unconstitutional in most advanced countries."[3] The policy adopted in the past by all countries where private insurance is sold is not to deny insurers access to medical information but rather to require that the medical information be accurate and up to date and that underwriting decisions be based on sound actuarial assumptions. These same requirements of fairness are appropriate for the use of future genomic information as well.

NOTES

The opinions expressed in this article are those of the author. They are not necessarily shared by any insurer or the insurance industry in general.

1. H. T. Bailey, T. M. Hutchinson, G. R. Narber, "The Regulatory Challenge to Life Insurance Classification," *Drake Law Review Insurance Annual* 25 (1976).

2. *Record of the Society of Actuaries,* San Francisco Meeting, 14–15 June 1990, 16:3 (1990): 1362.

3. "Ethics and the Human Genome," *Nature* 351 (1991): 591.

7

THE GENOME PROJECT, INDIVIDUAL DIFFERENCES, AND JUST HEALTH CARE

Norman Daniels

The mapping of the human genome is likely to have important implications for the just distribution of health care services. Some of these implications will be the result of the new medical technologies that will be developed once we learn more about the human genome. Despite their likely importance, I will not speculate about them in what follows, nor will I comment on the way they add to the burden we already have in deciding how to disseminate and ration new technologies under conditions of resource scarcity. Instead, I want to focus on the fact that the mapping of the genome will give us specific, new *information about individual variation.* This information can be used in good and bad, fair and unfair ways, and it raises, or rather refocuses, important questions about how we should distribute health care resources.

I shall address three sets of questions of genuine philosophical interest, each of which is sharpened in some way by what we learn about human variation from the genome project. One probable outcome of the genome project is a greater ability to predict certain health risks as a result of genetic screening. We will better be able to divide people into risk groups, not only for strictly genetic diseases but also for other diseases that have some genotypic component. This predictive ability may lead to better preventive or treatment regimens, but it is also of interest to private insurers who may want to use the information to exclude some individuals from insurance and to facilitate the risk rating of insurance pools. The ethical question posed by the underwriting practices of insurers is this: are people at lower risk entitled to benefit (through better access to cheaper insurance) from this sort of individual variation? More generally, which variations among individuals should be the basis for gaining advantage over others and which variations should we treat as a collective asset or liability? This first set of questions take us deep into political philosophy.

The second question is this: can we defend the distinction between medical therapies that *treat* and those that *enhance* in the face of new genetic information that allows us to pinpoint the genetic contributors to traits we want to alter? Imagine, for example, that we will come to identify particular genes or patterns of genes that contribute to making people very short. (I say "imagine" advisedly, since all interesting traits are highly heterogeneous; in what follows, we indulge in some of the fanciful expectations advanced by human genome proponents.) These genes do not represent pathology of the usual sort; for example, they do not lead to growth hormone deficiency. But being able to look at the microstructure underlying the "normal" distribution of height may produce strong pressures to identify a new class of "bad genes" and to suggest that people who have those genes now have a claim on others to assist them in changing their traits. These questions thus have vast implications for resource allocation. Like the preceding questions, they also take us deep into political philosophy. What we are really asking is which inequalities among people give rise to claims on others and which are matters of individual responsibility.

Finally, a question I shall discuss only briefly and largely by way of warning is this: how will new information that some individuals are at higher risk for disease, because of their genotype, affect our assumptions about responsibility for health and disease? For example, although we already know that "family history" has a bearing on susceptibility to heart disease or cancer, we also insist that people take responsibility for smoking, alcohol consumption, diet, and exercise, which also constitute risk factors. Will having much more specific information about genotype encourage acceptance of genetic determinism, undermining our current emphasis on responsibility for preventive health measures? Or will it increase the burden of responsibility we impose on those who are genotypically at greatest risk? Will we share the burden of making environments as conducive to good health as possible, drawing the lesson from the genome project that we all face some genotypically increased risks? How will these changes in our attitude toward responsibility affect our beliefs about our obligations to provide medical services?

As we shall see, none of these questions arises solely because of the new information we gather from the genome project. Each is already an issue for us. But quantity sometimes has qualitative effects, and the prevalence of contexts forcing these questions on us will increase as a result of what we learn about human variation from the genome project.

ACTUARIAL FAIRNESS AND INDIVIDUAL DIFFERENCES: ARE HEALTH RISKS INDIVIDUAL ASSETS OR COLLECTIVE BURDENS?

Suppose that one outcome of the genome project is the development of various screening tests that allow us to predict who is at higher risk for a variety of medical conditions. These tests could be used to extend what I shall refer to as *standard underwriting practices:* denying coverage, or offering more expensive and substandard coverage, to those who have a disease or at higher risk of contracting it in the future, as determined by various medical examinations, tests, records, or other "predictors" of risk. Is there a sound moral justification for these practices?[1]

The best strategy for insurers would be to develop a knock-down argument that showed we are *morally required* to use standard underwriting practices. Such an argument would seize the high moral ground and not simply rest on an appeal to their economic interest. Seeking such an argument, some insurers argue that it is *actuarially unfair,* and therefore morally unfair, to those at low medical risk when insurers do not exclude those at high risk from insurance pools. Thus, the hybrid term *actuarial fairness,* widely used in the literature, expresses the *moral* judgment that *fair underwriting* practices must reflect the division of people according to the *actuarially accurate* determination of their risks. I shall refer to this as "the argument from actuarial fairness."

Let us begin by thinking solely about the risk management aspect of medical insurance, ignoring for the moment any special moral importance we may attribute to ensuring access to health care services. From this perspective, health insurance is only a way for rational economic agents to manage their risks of serious losses under conditions of uncertainty. Prudent people buy insurance because they prefer to face modest losses (premiums) on a regular basis rather than face catastrophic losses at unpredictable times. The absence of information about when losses will occur gives people an interest in pooling risks. When all parties symmetrically lack information, prudent consumers of insurance will have a common interest in sharing their risks.

The situation changes when we acquire information that allows us to disaggregate the risk and sort people into stratified risk pools. For example, suppose we can differentiate risks by using information about the construction, age, density, and location of houses, as well as information about available firefighting facilities and relevant fire safety codes. Or suppose we can differentiate risks through information about individual medical histories, genetic disposition to disease or genetic disorders,[2] or lifestyle choices, such as smoking. Then, those purchasing insurance will come to see themselves as having distinct rather than common interests. Those at lower risk will prefer to pool their risks only with others at comparably low risk, since that will lower the cost of buying security. They may not want to subsidize security for those at higher risk. At the same time, those at high risk will seek the bargain in security offered by insurance that pools high and low risk individuals together; those at greatest risk need the insurance the most and seek it out. (This is called adverse selection.)

If they are to remain competitive, insurers must respond to these consumer preferences. They must protect themselves against adverse selection, excluding those at higher risk; they can then aggressively market insurance to those at lower risk who seek security at a lower price. The behavior of insurers thus responds to competitive forces *in a particular marketing context,* one that assumes health insurance has the primary function of giving individuals the opportunity to manage risks prudently.[3] This assumption, as we shall see, is far from morally neutral. Changing the rules governing insurance marketing, for example, by making insurance compulsory or by requiring that all insurance be community rated, would not eliminate the profit from insurance. But justifying those changes requires a different assumption about the function of insurance—that insurance is necessary to guarantee people adequate access to medical care.

The concept of actuarial fairness could be assigned a purely *de-*

scriptive as opposed to *normative* content in the kind of "risk management" insurance market we have just been considering. Saying that a premium is "actuarially fair" would mean only that it reflects the actuarial risks the purchaser faces, in other words, that it is actuarially *accurate*. The appeal to actuarial fairness that we find in the insurance literature goes beyond this purely descriptive content, however, and carries the implication that actuarially accurate underwriting practices are also morally fair or just ones. Insurers thus defend standard underwriting practices by claiming that

> insurance is founded on the principle that policyholders with the same expected risk of loss should be treated equally ... The primary goal of underwriting is the accurate prediction of future mortality and morbidity costs. An insurance company has the *responsibility* to treat all its policyholders *fairly* by establishing premiums at a level consistent with the risk represented by each individual policyholder.[4]

Specifically, it would be unfair to those at low risk if they are made to pay the higher premiums necessary to cover the costs of those at high risk. The remark about the "responsibility" of insurers suggests that it is an *obligation* to refuse to underwrite those at high risk.

The argument from actuarial fairness confuses *actuarial fairness* with *moral fairness* or *just distribution*. These are different notions: actuarial fairness is neither a necessary nor a sufficient condition for moral fairness or justice in an insurance scheme, especially in a health insurance scheme. To forge the link this argument does between fairness and actuarial fairness presupposes that individuals are entitled to benefit from *any* of their individual differences, especially their different risks for disease and disability. This presupposition is not only highly controversial, it is false.

To get from the merely descriptive notion of actuarial fairness, which has no justificatory force, to the moral claim about fairness found in the insurer's argument, we need to add some moral assumptions. Specifically, we have to add the *strong* assumption that individuals should be free to pursue the economic advantage that derives from any of their individual traits, including their proneness to disease and disability. The strong assumption might be used in an argument that echoes some recent work on distributive justice. First, individual differences—any individual differences—constitute some of an individual's personal assets. Second, people should be free to, indeed are entitled to, gain advantages from any of their personal assets. Third, social arrangements will be just only if they respect such liberties and entitlements. And fourth, specifically, individuals are entitled to have markets, including medical insurance markets, structured in such a way that they can pursue the advantages that can derive from their personal assets.

This skeletal argument can be elaborated, and the strong assumption it contains be defended (or attacked), in quite different ways within different theories of justice. For example, Nozick's libertarianism begins with certain assumptions about property rights and the degree to which certain liberties, such as the liberty to exchange one's marketable abilities or traits for personal advantage, must be respected even in the face of what many take to be overriding social goals.[5] Consequently, actuarially unfair schemes confiscate property without consent. Other political philosophers claim that just arrangements are the result of a bargain made by rational people who want to divide the benefits of mutual cooperation.[6] On this view, bargainers who have initial advantages in assets would only accept social arrangements that retain their relative advantages. As a result, bargainers might argue that just arrangements would preserve the advantages of those at low risk of disease through insurance markets that use standard underwriting practices.

An important objection to both libertarian and bargaining approaches is that the significant inequalities such theories justify can be traced back to initial inequalities for which there is little moral justification. To avoid this problem, Rawls imagines a "hypothetical contract" made by "free" and "equal" moral agents who are kept from knowing anything about their individual traits; they must select principles of justice that would work to everyone's advantage, including those who are worst off. Just which individual differences should be allowed to yield individual advantage thus becomes a matter for deliberation within the theory of justice, not a starting point for it.[7] We now need an argument for why this model for selecting principles is fair to all people and why we should count its outcome as justified, since we can no longer claim they are justified by appealing to the interests of actual property holders or bargainers.[8]

The debate about the relevance of individual differences to the just distributions of social goods thus touches on deep issues about equality that lie at the heart of the conflict between alternative approaches to constructing and justifying theories of justice. Showing that the strong assumption about individual differences is deeply controversial at the level of the theory of justice is obviously not a refutation of the argument from actuarial fairness. Still, we now have good reason not to accept the assumption without a convincing argument.

As it stands, the strong assumption is much too strong. Some individual differences are ones we clearly think should not be allowed to yield advantage or disadvantage. In recent legislation in the United States, we have established a legal framework to reinforce these views about justice. For example, we believe that race or sex should not become a basis for advantage or disadvantage in the distribution of rights, liberties, opportunities, or economic gain, even though these traits carry with them market advantage and disadvantage. Thus, we reject, in its most general form, the view that all individual differences can be a moral basis for advantage or disadvantage.

Although we agree that race and sex are clearly unacceptable bases for advantage, we have less agreement about how to treat some other individual differences. We allow talents and skills, for example, to play a role in the generation of inequalities, and yet we tax those with the most highly rewarded talents and skills in ways that help those who lack them, at least to some extent. (Rawls asks for a redistribution or tax that makes those who are worst off as well as they can be; this goes beyond what we do in practice.) How much inequality we allow is controversial in practice, just as it is in theory. Some people, like Nozick, think that individuals are entitled to derive whatever advantages the market allows from their talents and skills, and they view income redistribution as an unjustifiable tax on talents and skills. Others, like Rawls, argue that talents and skills, such as intelligence or manual dexterity, are the results of a "natural lottery," and that it is a matter of luck, not desert, who enjoys the family and social structures that encourage traits of character such as diligence necessary to refine one's basic talents. On this view, redistributive schemes are a morally obligatory form of social insurance that protects us against turning out to be among those who are worst off with regard to marketable talents and skills.

Even among those philosophers who want to treat talents and skills as individual assets, only the strictest libertarians treat health status differences merely as "unfortunate" variations and believe that there is no social obligation to correct for the relative advantages and disadvantages caused by disease or disability.[9] The design of health care systems throughout most of the world rests on a rejection of the view that individuals should have the opportunity to gain economic advantage from differences in their health risks. Despite variations in how these societies distribute the premium and tax burdens of financing universal health care insurance, the mixed system of the United States is nearly unique in allowing the degree of risks to play such a role. Far from being a self-evident or intuitively obvious moral principle, the strong assumption is widely rejected, both in theory and practice.

Two further points about the practice of insurers and society strengthen the claim that we do not in fact treat actuarial fairness as a basic principle of distributive justice. If insurers thought it were such a basic principle, we might expect that they would try to develop and use all possible information about variations in risk among insurees. But insurers use information about risks only when it is in *their economic interest* to do so. In effect, the principle actually underlying their practice is that we are entitled to benefit from our differences only if the market makes it profitable for insurers to provide such benefits.

This market-based entitlement can be construed as a principle of fairness only if we think the market is a fair procedure for drawing the distinctions we want to make. But, and this is the second point, we do not trust the market to draw the distinctions we think it is fair to make in this regard. We *override* appeals to actuarial fairness for many reasons in both medical and nonmedical insurance contexts. For example, we condemned "redlining" in the late 1970s as an unacceptable underwriting practice, although no one questioned its utility as a (rough) predictor of risks of loss. (A "red line" was drawn around a particular geographical area and its (largely minority) residents were then excluded from insurance or mortgages.) Similarly, unisex rating is a rejection of an actuarially fair and efficient method of underwriting and pricing groups at differential risk, but we here override standard underwriting practices because we give more importance to a principle of distributive justice ensuring equal treatment of groups that are the traditional targets of discrimination. Similarly, some states have established insurance pools that guarantee no one is deemed uninsurable because of prior medical condition or high risk classification. Where such pools are funded by insurance premiums paid by low risk individuals, we simply have an enforced "subsidy" from those at low risk to those at high risk, overriding concerns about actuarial fairness. Our practice shows that we do not believe that actuarial fairness is a basic requirement of justice.

There is, however, a more compelling argument for rejecting the view that health insurance must be structured so that individuals can derive benefits from their differences in medical risks. Health care does many things for people: it extends life, reduces suffering, provides information and assurance, and in other ways improves the quality of life. Nevertheless, it has one general function of overriding importance for purposes of justice: it maintains, restores, or compensates for the loss of—in short, protects—functioning that is normal for a member of our species. Normal functioning is a crucial determinant of the opportunities open to an individual since disease or disability shrink the range of opportunities that would otherwise have been available to someone with particular talents and skills in a given society. Since justice requires that we protect *fair equality of opportunity* for individuals in a society, it requires that we design health care institutions, including their method of reimbursement, so that they protect opportunity as well as possible within reasonable limits on resources.[10] Specifically, justice requires that there be no financial barriers to access to care and that the system allocate its limited resources so that they work effectively to protect normal functioning and thus fair equality of opportunity. In fact, we get a rough way to assess the importance of particular health care services, namely, by their effect on the normal opportunity range. Any general theory of justice that includes a strong principle protecting fair equality of opportunity will be able to incorporate my account of justice and health care.

The view I have been sketching involves rejecting the argument from actuarial fairness. A health care system is just provided that it protects fair equality of opportunity. Our system uses standard underwriting practices, but it fails to protect equal opportunity since access to care depends on ability to pay. Therefore, these underwriting practices are not a sufficient condition for ensuring that the system is just. It will be clear from what follows that these practices are not a necessary condition either.

The most common way to try to meet social obligations regarding access to health care is to institute a universal, compulsory national health insurance scheme. Under social insurance schemes, prior medical conditions and risk classification cannot serve as the basis for underwriting or pricing insurance coverage. Rather, because society acts on its obligation to meet all reasonable health care needs, within limits on resources, there will be subsidies from the well to the ill and from low risk to high risk individuals, as well as from the rich to the poor. The social insurance scheme thus *requires* what a private market for health insurance would condemn as actuarially unfair. This point is independent of whether the national health insurance scheme includes a sector with private insurance. The German and Dutch systems, for example, have many private insurers, but they are prohibited from using standard underwriting practices.

From the perspective of a private insurer in our mixed system, denying coverage to those at high risk seems completely unproblematic ("you cannot buy fire insurance once the engines are on the way"). But this perspective is persuasive only if the central function of health insurance is risk management. Since health insurance has a different social function—protecting equality of opportunity by guaranteeing access to an appropriate array of medical services—then there is a clear *mismatch* between standard underwriting practices and the social function of health insurance. A just, purely public health insurance system thus leaves no room for the notion of actuarial fairness.

Ironically, a just but mixed public and private health insurance system makes actuarial fairness a largely *illusory*, perhaps even deceptive, notion. Suppose that high risk individuals, such as those with a history of high blood pressure, are excluded from private insurance schemes in a mixed insurance system, for the kinds of reasons noted earlier. Since the system is just, however, these people will not be left uninsured, as many are in the United States today. They will be covered by public insurance or by legally mandated high risk insurance pools subsidized by premiums from private insurance. Those lower risk individuals left in the private insurance schemes might think that actuarial fairness has protected them from higher premiums. But here is where their savings are largely illusory. The premiums of those in the private insurance schemes will either cross-subsidize the high risk individuals who are insured in the special high risk pools, or their taxes will cover the costs of insuring high risk individuals through public schemes. Their actual insurance premiums are thus their private ones plus the share of their taxes that goes to public insurance.

The main point of principle in a just mixed system is this: low risk individuals still share the burden of financing the health risks of high risk individuals. Fairness requires that these risks be shared, not, as the argument from actuarial fairness would have it, that they not be. In effect, health risks are not treated as economic assets and liabilities for the individual.

The human genome project will generate information that insurers in our system will want to use in standard underwriting practices, not because they are greedy but because they respond to the incentives we have built into the design of our system. The argument I have offered says that such uses will make our system *less fair* and *more unjust.* But the problem is not that new information will emerge from the genome project. In a national health insurance scheme that prohibits our morally unacceptable underwriting practices, information about risks would not be used to exclude people from treatment but rather to improve counseling, education, and treatment. It is not the availability of the information that is bad but rather how our system forces us to use it. If we fail to correct the more basic injustice in the health care system, then singling out information from the genome project for special treatment would itself seem arbitrary. The problem must be corrected at its source—the design of our health care system—not simply where a new symptom of the injustice arises.

CAN WE RETAIN THE TREATMENT VERSUS ENHANCEMENT DISTINCTION?

We have social obligations to treat disease and disability because of their impact on opportunity, and so we should not accept the barriers to access that follow from standard underwriting practices. Are these obligations limited to treating disease and disability? Or does any condition that creates an inequality in opportunity for welfare or advantage among individuals give rise to claims on others? In rejecting the argument from actuarial fairness, we countered an attack from the right on our social obligations to treat disease and disability. I want to consider now an attack from the left on the way I have formulated these obligations. The attack rests on the view that our egalitarian concerns require us to eliminate inequalities among people that arise from many conditions other than disease and disability. In effect, it is a demand for a more radical version of equality of opportunity. In the context of health care, the attack takes the form of a challenge to the distinction between treatment and enhancement.

I suggested earlier that the genome project may provide us with information that will erode the distinction we often draw between uses of medical technology for treatment of disease and disability and uses that enhance human appearance or performance. This distinction is closely connected to the frequently used, but poorly understood, concept of "medical necessity." Many public and private insurance schemes in the United States (and Canada) claim to provide only medically necessary services: many services that involve only enhancement (such as "cosmetic" surgery) are thus excluded from coverage on these grounds. I shall suggest in what follows that the treatment versus enhancement distinction does have a moral justification, at least relative to a *standard* way of thinking about equality of opportunity. The genetic information about human variation provided by the genome project may make that distinction seem more arbitrary, and to the extent that it does, it poses a challenge to the standard model and the use to which I have put it in thinking about justice and health care. Of course, this is not a conceptually novel threat; viewed from the perspective of the attack from the left, the distinction and the standard model it depends on already seem arbitrary. But the new information may heighten the appearance of moral arbitrariness, and that is the reason for discussing the issue here.

Many medical technologies, new and old, can alter people in ways they desire to be changed. When do we have a social obligation to ensure that such preferences are met? Do rights to health care include entitlements to have those preferences met, resources permitting? What should insurance cover?

The most inclusive answer to these questions would be that we have such obligations whenever someone desires to eliminate an unwanted physical or mental condition. This would allow "subjective" preferences to place enormous demands on resources, making everyone hostage to the extravagant tastes of everyone else.[11] Since we generally do not believe it is medicine's task to make everyone equally happy, we reject this view and its implication that we should have to pay for liposuction or face lifts. Instead, we think obligations arise only when medical treatments address more important problems. The stance we thus take about medicine is compatible with rejecting, as Rawls and Dworkin do, a broad form of egalitarianism that would require us to ensure the equal welfare or happiness of all individuals.[12]

A less inclusive answer would be that we have obligations to provide medical care whenever people desire to eliminate conditions that put them at some disadvantage. The notion of disadvantage is meant to be objective, including some forms of suffering as well as the competitive disadvantages that result from the lack of capabilities, such as marketable talents or skills. This view has some initial moral appeal when the disadvantages are not our fault or the (even unlucky) result of our prior choices. Our egalitarian inclinations may incline us to think we owe something toward eliminating them.[13] If we adopt such a radical view—the left position I referred to earlier—we may have to assign medicine a much greater a role as a social equalizer than we now assign it. At least currently, it is not medicine's task to make everyone an equal competitor, wherever possible eliminating all inequalities in the distribution of talents and skills or other capabilities.[14]

A more modest answer, one that tends to match a wide range of our practices, including our insurance practices, is that we have obligations to provide services whenever someone desires that a medical *need* be met. Generally, this is taken to mean that the service involves *treatment of a disease or disability,* where disease and disability are seen as departures from species-typical normal functional organization or functioning.[15] Characterizing medical need in this way implies a contrast between uses of medical services that *treat* disease (or disability) conditions and uses that merely *enhance* human performance or appearance. Enhancement does not meet a medical need even where the service may correct for a competitive disadvantage that does not result from prior choices. Accordingly, medicine has the role of making people *normal* competitors, not *equal* competitors; this role fits, I shall claim, with the standard model for thinking about equality of opportunity.

Despite its wide appeal, the distinction between treatment and enhancement may seem arbitrary in light of hard cases such as these:

Johnny is a short 11-year-old boy with documented GH [growth hormone] deficiency resulting from a brain tumor. His parents are of average height. His predicted adult height without GH treatment is approximately 160 cm (5 feet 3 inches).

Billy is a short 11-year-old boy with normal GH secretion according to current testing methods. However, his parents are extremely short, and he has a predicted adult height of 160 cm (5 feet 3 inches).[16]

These cases make the distinction seem arbitrary for several reasons. First, Johnny and Billy will suffer disadvantage equally if they are not treated. There is no reason to think the difference in the underlying causes of their shortness will lead people to treat them in ways that make one happier or more advantaged than the other. Second, although Johnny is short because of dysfunction whereas Billy is short because of his (normal) genotype, both are short through no choice or fault of their own. The shortness is in both cases the result of a biological "natural lottery." Both thus seem to suffer undeserved disadvantages. Third, Billy's preference for greater height, just like Johnny's, is a preference that most people hold; it is not peculiar, idiosyncratic, or extravagant. Indeed, it is a response to a social prejudice, "heightism." The prejudice is what we should condemn, not the fact that they both form an "expensive taste" in reaction to it.

Cases such as these raise the following question: does the concept of disease underlying the treatment versus enhancement distinction force us to treat relevantly similar cases in dissimilar ways? Are we violating the old Aristotelian requirement that justice requires treating like cases similarly? Is dissimilar treatment unfair or unjust?

Despite the challenge of hard cases, the treatment versus enhancement distinction should play a role in deciding what obligations we have to provide medical services. To show that this distinction is not arbitrary from the viewpoint of justice, despite the hard cases, I shall argue that it fits better than do alternatives with what I call the *standard model* for thinking about equality of opportunity. Of course, the standard model may itself be indefensible, a point I will return to shortly. First, though, I want to show that the standard model helps specify a reasonable limit on the central task of health care.

Earlier I noted that disease and disability restrict the range of opportunities open to an individual. Health care services maintain, restore, and compensate for losses of function that result from disease and disability. They thus restore people to the range of capabilities they *could be expected to have had* without disease or disability, given their allotment of talents and skills. Our *standard model* for thinking about equality of opportunity thus depends on *taking as a given the fact that talents and skills and other capabilities are not distributed equally* among people. Some people are better at some things than others. Accordingly, we ensure people *fair* equality of opportunity if we judge them by their capabilities while ignoring "morally irrelevant" traits such as sex or race when we place people in schools, jobs, and offices. Often, however, we must correct for cases in which capabilities have been misdeveloped through racist, sexist, or other discriminatory practices. Similarly, by preventing or treating disease and disability, we can correct for impairment of the capabilities people would otherwise have. The standard model does not call for eliminating differences in normal capabilities in general, let alone through medical enhancement.

This limitation of the standard model can appear arbitrary. As I noted earlier, our capabilities are themselves the result of a natural and social lottery, and we do not "deserve" them. We just are fortunate or unfortunate in having them. We can mitigate this underlying arbitrariness somewhat as follows. Those who are better endowed with marketable capabilities are likely to enjoy more goods such as income, wealth, and power. If we constrain inequalities in these goods so that those who are worst off do as well as possible, considering all alternatives, then social cooperation will work to the benefit of all.[17] Still, this constraint does not eliminate all inequalities in the individual capabilities or in the resulting opportunities individuals enjoy, especially since we are enjoined to judge people by their capabilities and not by their "morally irrelevant" traits such as sex or race. If our egalitarian concerns require that we strive to give people equal capabilities, wherever technologically feasible, then we should not settle for mitigating the effects of the normal distribution of capabilities, as proponents of the standard model of equality of opportunity would have it.[18] Rejecting the standard model pushes us toward equalizing all differences in capabilities; from that perspective, the distinction between treatment and enhancement has no point, at least where enhancement is aimed at equalizing capabilities.

Information from the genome project might make the distinction between disease (including genetic disease) and the normal distribution of capabilities seem more arbitrary. Suppose we learn that some particular pattern of genes explains the extreme shortness of Billy, the child who was not deficient in growth hormone. That is, we learn just which "losing numbers" in the natural lottery placed Billy in the bottom one percent of the normal distribution for height. Identifying these genes may then tempt us to think of them as "bad" ones: they lead to Billy's unhappiness or disadvantage in a "heightist" world. We will then be sorely tempted to think of them very much on the model of genetic defects or diseases, especially if they work through mechanisms that have some analogy to pathological defects. In other words, we will be tempted to medicalize what we have hitherto considered normal. What, after all, allows us to treat the "bad genes" differently from genes that lead to growth hormone deficiency or to receptor insensitivity to grown hormone? If we can remedy the effects of these genes with growth hormone treatment or other treatments, including genetic tampering, we might think it quite arbitrary to maintain the treatment versus enhancement distinction.

I want to offer several points as a limited defense of the standard model and the treatment versus enhancement distinction. Both versions of equality of opportunity, the standard model and the more radical one that requires equalizing capabilities, seem to appeal to the same underlying intuition—that advantages and disadvantages resulting from the natural lottery are not themselves deserved. But they use the intuition differently. The standard model suggests we mitigate the effects of normally distributed capabilities through restrictions on other inequalities we allow. Since some inequality in capabilities is a fact of life, the task is to mitigate their effects while adopting principles that let everyone benefit from social cooperation. The criticism from the left rests far more weight on the underlying intuition: it says that wherever possible we must actually try to reduce variance in the distribution of capabilities, equalizing them wherever possible. I believe that the standard model better captures our actual concerns about equality than the more radical version. (Of course, our actual concerns may be too limited, so this is not a conclusive argument.)

Some supporting evidence for this point derives from our moral beliefs and practices concerning health care. We regard medical services as meeting *urgent needs* when they are aimed at restoring or maintaining "normal functioning." Our consensus about where to draw the line focuses on eliminating disease and disability. We already have many technologies that can enhance functioning for individuals, even giving them advantages (such as beauty or athletic performance) they previously did not have. But we generally resist assimilating these cases of enhancement to cases of treatment because we do not see them as meeting important needs. Although these enhancing services alter traits that may be the results of a natural lottery, they involve optimizing capabilities that are not departures from normal functional organization or functioning.

Of course, what makes the case of Billy and Johnny problematic is that they both suffer equal disadvantage as a result of the natural lottery (and social prejudice). But there is justification for adhering to a distinction that captures and sustains social agreement on important matters, even if the distinction seems arbitrary in isolated hard cases. The line between treatment and enhancement is generally uncontroversial and ascertainable through publicly accepted methods, such as those of the biomedical sciences. Being able to draw a line in this way allows us to refer counterfactually in a relatively clear and objective way to the range of opportunities a person *would have had* in the absence of disease and disability; it facilitates public agreement. Because of these virtues, not every hard case counts as a counterexample that warrants overturning the distinction.

The "equal capabilities" approach, bolstered by new information from the genome project, is likely to undermine agreement on the importance of meeting medical needs. According to it, we would now have many more such needs, for much of what we now take to be normal would become conditions in need of rectification. Since we are far less likely to think that it is "urgent" to correct the effects of these newly labeled "bad genes," shifting away from the standard model is likely to undermine consensus on the moral importance of health care.

Will it be possible to hold the line? Some relief may come from a more careful attempt to examine the distinction between genetic disease and normal variation. This may enable us to offer a theoretical justification, coming out of the biological sciences, for a baseline distinction. It is important to note that I am not trying to save the appeal to a natural baseline here because there is something magical or metaphysically basic about it. Nor am I violating Hume's injunction against deriving "ought" from "is." Rather, the natural baseline both facilitates and reflects moral agreement about the urgency of medical care. I also believe there is moral justification for limiting in some ways the task involved in protecting equality of opportunity, otherwise it will be discredited as too demanding an ideal. If, however, no theoretical justification is forthcoming that lets us distinguish "bad" (or nonoptimal) genes from genetic disease, then we will have to give more complex justifications for drawing the line between cases in which we have obligations to provide services and those in which we do not. My claim is simply that it will be harder to reach consensus on these justifications without the ability to appeal to a natural baseline, however imperfectly drawn.

I have been offering reasons not to expand our goals in protecting equality of opportunity from the more limited ones of the standard model to the more encompassing one of equalizing capabilities. Nevertheless, our obligations to provide medical services need not derive solely from the concerns about equality of opportunity that I have argued are central. For example, I think we have compelling reasons for providing public funding of nontherapeutic abortions that go beyond their importance for preventive health care. Similarly, suppose an inexpensive treatment became available for improving cognitive capabilities in childhood; administering it would greatly enhance the results of education, close the gap between poor but "normal" students and others, and contribute greatly to social productivity. We might then have compelling reasons to seek enhancement in this way, even if they differ from our standard justification for the importance of health care. Of course, we already have excellent reasons for putting more resources into education, yet we do not, despite the fact that our failure to do so results in misdeveloped talents and skills along race and class lines.

GENES AND RESPONSIBILITY FOR HEALTH

We now acknowledge that lifestyle choices about diet, exercise, and drug and alcohol abuse play a significant role in our risks for cardiovascular disease, cancer, and other diseases. Throughout the last decade, a cult of health fitness has gripped millions of Americans, although it is more prominent among the better-off socioeconomic groups. There is significant media and peer pressure to reduce smoking, alcohol consumption, and fat in diets, all around the theme of "taking responsibility for health." No doubt this movement will reduce the health risks for many people, and it is therefore beneficial on the whole. But the genome project is likely to reveal to us many unsuspected genetic influences on the risks for major "lifestyle" diseases, including addictions. It will then be the case that some people who have low risk genotypes can engage with few ill effects in what would be highly risky lifestyle choices for others. For example, some people who smoke may be more susceptible to addiction than others; among those who smoke, some may be more susceptible to lung cancer or other diseases than others. Conversely, people who follow low risk regimens with nearly religious fervor may reduce their risks only marginally if they have genotypes that predispose them to be at higher risk for these conditions. What are we to say about "responsibility for health" when the effects of responsible action are so varied?

As genetic information becomes more available, it is likely to have two effects on motivation. Some people may think that the risks they face are really "in the cards" and that there is little point to making life less pleasant when there is only a modest effect for them on overall risks. Others will draw the opposite conclusion: it will become imperative for them to devote extra effort to reducing the high risks they face. Their genes have put the ball in their court. It is difficult to say which of these effects on motivation will be greater, but there is some chance that public concern with taking responsibility for lifestyle choices will be reduced or fragmented by the discovery of significant genetic components. Similarly, our motivation to clean up the workplace, protecting workers against hazardous materials, may be reduced if we learn that some people are genotypically more sensitive to those hazards than others; we might then think it simply better to remove the more sensitive individuals from the workplace.[19] If new information coming from the genome project builds—deliberately or inadvertently—public belief in genetic determinism, then it is more likely that people will feel there is little they can do to protect themselves or susceptible workers. Unfortunately, as Richard Lewontin has noted, in their enthusiasm to promote the genome project, many of those with intellectual or economic interests in its success have said misleading things that promote beliefs in genetic determinism.[20]

There are corollary judgments third parties will make about responsibility. Some will see the presence of a large genetic influence on risks as an excusing condition. People who do little to modify their high risks will be excused on the grounds that there is really little they can do. Their best efforts will not reduce their risks to the levels faced by those with "good" genes who can eat, drink, and be merry at low risk. After all, how can we expect people to remain committed to being responsible for their health when so much of the effect is out of their hands? Others will say that the obligation to reduce risks is even greater for those whose genotype puts them at higher risk. It is bad enough that their genes place higher burdens on them and others; it is even worse if they know they impose those burdens and do not do what they can to reduce them. That is, there is a strong temptation to blame the victim. (As with the effects on motivation, there are also corresponding changes in third-party attitudes toward occupational hazards.)

Two issues of policy may emerge. First, the appearance of information about genotypic contributions may tend to fragment the public concern about responsibility for health. This is a bad effect we must try to counter. We should preserve and broaden the movement that encourages people to adopt healthy lifestyle choices and that will mean educating people carefully so that the new information about genotype does not reinforce belief in genetic determinism. Health risks are *phenotypic:* they result from the interaction of genotype and environment, including our lifestyle choices. Even strong genotypic effects can be countered by crucial environmental interventions (such as changing diet to reduce the effects of phenylketonuria). Though the urgency of this message may differ for people with different genotypes, and though the incentives may vary as well, there is still an effect of lifestyle choices that will have to be carefully documented and made the basis of continuing education and even incentives, such as through discounts on life insurance. Of course, the effort to retain such incentives will be set back if genetic screening for life insurance produces a different set of rewards and punishments.

Second, there may be a reduction in the temptation to blame those who become ill from diseases for which there is a significant lifestyle component. This would be a positive effect of new genetic information about human variation, a modest reduction in the temptation to blame the victim. We would be less tempted to look at anyone with coronary artery disease or even alcoholism as paying the price for their lifestyle sins. We would be in a weaker position to resent the burdens they impose on us since they may have been at higher risk than average no matter what their lifestyle choices. Whether this positive effect emerges, however, depends on facts about the structure of our health care system. If we retain a private insurance sector that is free to engage in standard underwriting practices, then, for the reasons discussed earlier, economic forces will work against our willingness to share risks and the burdens of disease collectively.

CONCLUSIONS

I have argued for the following specific answers to the three questions raised by new information about individual variation. First, although we may better predict which individuals are prone to certain diseases, and thus which individuals are worse insurance risks, justice requires that we not use this information in ways that make it more difficult for such people to obtain appropriate health care. This means we should revamp our insurance system so that it does not exclude those at high risk from adequate coverage. Drawing this conclusion required showing that individuals are not entitled to benefit economically from all their genetically based advantages. Second, despite the fact that new information about genotypes may throw light on the genetic factors contributing to below average (but still normal) appearance or function, we can still draw a plausible distinction between treatment and enhancement and give priority to medical treatments rather than enhancements. That is, we can still uphold a rationing principle we currently employ. Third, we should not be mislead into accepting genetic determinism, for doing so may undermine our support for plausible beliefs about responsibility for health. Finding out that some people are genotypically more susceptible to diseases that also have a lifestyle component does not imply that we should ignore the effect of environment on phenotype.

Some general points deserve emphasis, by way of conclusion. None of these questions is truly novel: each is raised by current practices, independently of the human genome project. Nevertheless, each is sharpened and made more urgent by information we obtain about the genome. The information we obtain from the genome project is by itself neither good nor bad; what we do with it determines its value. Better information about the risk of disease can lead to better prevention or treatment—or it can be used to exclude people from insurance. Better information about genetically increased risks can be used to focus attention on the importance or lifestyle choices; the information can be used to educate and support or to blame and punish. Finally, the structure of our institutions may incline us or tempt us to use the information for good or for bad purposes. An insurance system that endorses standard underwriting practices makes it look "natural" to place extra economic burdens on those at greater risk for disease; an insurance system that treats risks as a collective, not individual liability, does the opposite. Justice requires that we share certain risks, and so it behooves us to reform some of our institutions. Unfortunately, if we do not strive for just institutions, potentially useful information, such as that deriving from the genome project, is readily put to unjust purposes.

NOTES

Acknowledgment: This work was in part supported by the National Endowment for the Humanities (RH20917) and the National Library of Medicine (1RO1LM05005).

1. Norman Daniels, "Insurability and the HIV problem: Ethical Issues in Underwriting," *Milbank Quarterly* 68:4 (1990): 497–526.

2. S. E. Antonarkakis, "Diagnosis of Genetic Disorders at the DNA Level," *New England Journal of Medicine* 320 (1989): 153–161.

3. J. D. Hammond and A. F. Shapiro, "AIDS and the Limits of Insurability," *Milbank Quarterly* 64:1 (1986): 143–167.

4. K. A. Clifford and R. P. Iuculano, "AIDS and Insurance: The Rationale for AIDS-related testing, " *Harvard Law Review* 100(1987): 1807–1809. Emphasis added.

5. Robert Nozick, *Anarchy, State, and Utopia* (New York: Basic Books, 1974).

6. David Gauthier, *Morals by Agreement* (Oxford, U.K.: Oxford University Press, 1986)

7. John Rawls, *A Theory of Justice* (Cambridge, MA: Harvard University Press, 1971).

8. John Rawls, "Kantian Constructivism in Moral Theory," *Journal of Philosophy* 77:9(1980): 515–572. Also relevant is John Rawls, "Justice as Fairness: A Briefer Description" (unpubl. ms., 1989).

9. H. Tristam Engelhardt, Jr., *The Foundations of Bioethics* (New York: Oxford University Press, 1986).

10. Norman Daniels, *Just Health Care* (Cambridge, U.K.: Cambridge University Press, 1985).

11. John Rawls, "Social Unity and Primary Goods," In A. Sen and B. Williams, eds., *Utilitarianism and Beyond* (Cambridge, U.K.: Cambridge University Press, 1982), 159–186. See also Daniels, "Just Health Care," 23–25.

12. Rawls, "Social Unity." See also Ronald Dworkin, "What is Equality? Part I: Equality of Welfare," *Philosophy and Public Affairs* 10:3(1982): 185–246.

13. G. A. Cohen, "On the Currency of Egalitarian Justice," *Ethics* 99(1989): 906–944. See also R. J. Arneson, "Equality and Equal Opportunity for Welfare," *Philosophical Studies* 54(1988): 79–95.

14. Norman Daniels, "Equality of What: Welfare, Resources, or Capabilities?" *Philosophy and Phenomenological Research* 50(1990, supp.): 273–296.

15. Christopher Boorse, "Health as a Theoretical Concept," *Philosophy of Science* 44(1977): 542–573. See also Christopher Boorse, "On the Distinction Between Disease and Illness," *Philosophy and Public Affairs* 5:1(1975): 49–68.

16. D. B. Allen and N. C. Fost, "Growth Hormone Therapy for Short Stature: Panacea or Pandora's Box?" *Journal of Pediatrics* 117:1(1990): 16–21.

17. Rawls, *A Theory of Justice.*

18. A. Sen, "Justice: Means Versus Freedoms," *Philosophy and Public Affairs* 19 (1990): 111–121.

19. Daniels, *Just Health Care*, chap. 8.

20. Richard Lewontin, "The Dream of the Human Genome," *The New York Review of Books,* 28 May 1992, pp. 31–40.

8

JUST GENETICS
A Problem Agenda

Leonard M. Fleck

As I prepared to write this essay, the image that forced itself upon my mind was one of those ancient maps whose known world was framed with the words *Terra Incognita*. The more I considered the problem of justice in connection with emerging genetic technologies, the more I felt I was entering a territory that was largely unknown. Hence, this essay can be considered nothing more than a preliminary exploration of that territory. I shall feel that I have made a useful contribution if I can identify and articulate some of the distinctive problems of justice that are raised by the genetic technologies that are emerging in the wake of the human genome project.

It might be useful at this point to mention the major working hypotheses that are shaping this essay. First, many of these emerging genetic technologies cannot be thought of, morally speaking, as simply another advanced medical technology competing for resources in the medical marketplace. That is, if our society were to withdraw all research funding for the development of a totally implantable artificial heart, the result being that it would be very improbable that such a device would ever come into existence, we would have treated no one unjustly in our society. But I am inclined to argue that, at least for some emerging genetic technologies, this would not be true. That is, there are powerful considerations of justice that would require the development and dissemination of some emerging genetic technologies.[1]

Second, if is true that genetic technologies are not merely another medical technology without claim to moral priority, then perhaps we ought to think about this collection of moral issues in terms of a "sphere of genetic justice." Here I make an appeal to Michael Walzer's metaphor of "spheres of justice."[2] I think Walzer's pluralistic conception of justice represents a useful corrective to grand theories of justice that have a certain allure for philosophers. Deductive reasoning from any of these grand theories of justice will rarely yield moral resolution regarding, for example, problems of genetic justice. In other essays I have argued that there is a unique cast to problems of justice in the field of health care in general, and hence, we ought to think in terms of a *sphere of health care justice.*[3] Genetic justice might be seen as a subset of that larger sphere.

At this point, however, I should mention that I am less than comfortable with the sphere analogy, which suggests a neatness and isolation that is false to both our moral practice and an adequate conceptualization of health care justice. My preferred metaphor for genetic justice would be that of an urban neighborhood, which has rougher shifting boundaries and which is part of the urban megalopolis that is health care justice. There are lots of internal connections among the neighborhoods and suburbs that make up the megalopolis, which is to say that there are moral considerations that link up the neighborhoods of health care justice, but there are also distinctive qualities of the neighborhood or suburb that give it a character of its own. If I were to push the analogy one step further, then we might think of genetic justice as being a new suburb we are planning. Our choices are constrained by the street system and utilities that are adjacent, and by zoning, environmental, topological, and economic considerations, among others. But there is still room for considerable creativity with respect to the layout of that suburb, and the creative possibilities are enhanced by emerging building technologies. It is similarly the case with respect to the moral judgments and moral practices that will constitute our sense of genetic justice. The large-scale moral framework that seems most attuned to this analogy is that of Rawls' Kantian constructivism.[4] The slogan that best epitomizes this moral framework is that justice is political, not metaphysical.[5]

Third, philosophers have for the most part been enamoured with ideal conceptions of justice. There may be good logical and philosophical reasons why such debates are important, but these debates seem to do little by way of resolving concrete problems of medical or moral practice and public policy. From the perspective of ideal justice, all our public policy choices are morally flawed, and in some sense, unjust. A conclusion such as this is neither practically nor morally helpful. More accurately, it is pernicious if it encourages moral scepticism and indifference or arbitrariness. What I have argued for as an alternative are nonideal frameworks of justice.[6] This is what I believe is needed if we are to address intelligently and effectively the problems of genetic justice. When we adopt a nonideal framework, then we will be able to determine whether a specific resolution of a specific problem of genetic justice is "just enough." That is, we will be able to judge whether our proposed resolution justifiably represents a moral improvement over the current state of affairs, which is what often will be sufficient to warrant moral approbation.

One additional methodological point needs to be made. In moral practice, it is usually more difficult to achieve agreement on what justice *positively* requires of us regarding some redistribution of resources, as opposed to what justice *negatively* requires. That is, it seems easier to achieve agreement that a certain state of affairs is seriously unjust than to achieve agreement regarding the preferred just state of affairs that must replace the unjust state of affairs. For example, there is broad agreement among health economists, health policy analysts, and moral philosophers that the large tax subsidy we provide to the middle class for the purchase of health insurance benefits is seriously unjust. In 1992, this was a tax subsidy of about $64 billion, which is what federal and state governments would have collected in additional taxes if our health insurance had been taxed as income. The injustice is that seventy percent of those without health insurance in our society are working—but at low wage jobs that do not offer health insurance as a benefit. That means these individuals would have to purchase health insurance with after-tax dollars, which means their health insurance, if they could afford it, would have a forty percent premium attached to it. Yet these individuals, who are certainly less well off than the middle class, have helped to subsidize the middle class. It is difficult to imagine any conception of health care justice that would see this as a just state of affairs. The point here is that we should not minimize the moral importance of such negative moral agreement. If we can identify clear injustices with respect to the use or dissemination of emerging genetic technologies, then we will have made some moral progress.

Fourth, though the focus of this essay is on justice as a moral concern regarding emerging genetic technologies, the fact is that justice is not the only moral value that counts. One of the problems that has to be addressed is how we balance considerations of justice against other equally important moral considerations in this area. Again, my objective here will be to identify and map some of these moral conflicts as opposed to offering premature resolutions. In particular, I shall focus on possible conflicts between justice and liberalism regarding these emerging genetic technologies. Nozick and Rawls are generally viewed as offering diametrically opposed conceptions of justice, though in fact both offer what are described as "liberal" conceptions of justice. I take some of the essential features of a *liberal* conception of justice to be the following: (1) a strong emphasis on individual rights; (2) respect by the state for a zone of privacy and individual liberty marked out by these rights claims, a zone in which the state will not interfere and in which individuals can make choices regarding their lives in accord with their individual conceptions of the good; (3) official state neutrality with respect to competing conceptions of the good; and (4) state commitment to expanding the domain of liberty as much as is compatible with respect for the rights of all. As we shall see, there are a number of emerging genetic technological possibilities that will severely challenge the compatibility of liberalism and genetic justice.

JUSTICE AND EMERGING MEDICAL TECHNOLOGIES

After we have completed the task of mapping the human genome, would we be treating anyone unjustly if, say, we decided that no more research funds would be used to continue the development of a broad range of emerging genetic technologies? To make this scenario somewhat plausible, we could imagine that all the large health insurance companies in the United States had agreed that no policies would be issued that provided coverage for such technologies to be applied in health care settings; that would effectively squelch the profit motive. If the federal government endorsed this action as a way of gaining some control on escalating health costs, could the government be justifiably accused of having acted unjustly? There is considerable evidence to suggest that roughly half the problem of escalating health costs is attributable to these expensive emerging medical technologies.[7] Further, the claim might be advanced that no one really has a just claim to any of these emerging medical technologies, that it is a matter of social beneficence as to which, if any, of these technologies are nurtured and developed, and that so long as decisions about which technologies to support are not a product of obvious discriminatory judgment, no one has been treated unfairly.

In responding to the issue that has been raised, I want to begin by largely endorsing this last claim. That is, no one has been treated unjustly if, for example, society chooses not to develop a totally implantable artificial heart with the result that 350,000 people continue to die each year whose lives could have been extended by an additional five years if they had had access to that device. Having said that, however, I will also argue that at least some emerging genetic technologies belong in a special moral category because they do raise concerns of justice that must be explicitly addressed. Given limitations of space, we can only make some crude distinctions here, but they are still useful. We should distinguish, for example, emerging genetic testing technology from emerging gene therapy technology that is somatically focused from emerging germ-line genetic technology. Further, we should distinguish genetic tests that might be applied to adults for diagnostic purposes from those that might be applied to early fetuses from those that might be applied to four-cell embryos. For reasons that are explained later, I will argue that embryonic genetic testing and embryonic genetic engineering involve prima facie claims of justice.

What moral arguments can be given for saying that we, as a society, have not treated anyone unjustly if we refuse to provide any more funding for the development of a totally implantable artificial heart, the result being that such a device is likely never to be developed? If this means that 350,000 people each year will die from heart disease who otherwise would have had the opportunity for five extra years of life on average, then it seems that this ought to be cause for moral concern. However, I will argue that all these deaths might be unfortunate, as is true for any premature death, but not unjust. First, for all practical purposes, virtually all Americans are at risk for heart disease. Hence, failing to fund continued development of the totally implantable artificial heart does not represent arbitrary and unjustified discrimination against some identifiable group of individuals, as would be the case if a white-dominated society refused to provide any research funds for sickle cell anemia, or some other disease that was especially burdensome to some disfavored group. Second, individuals who suffer from heart disease have no special moral claims against society, as might be the case with coal miners who suffer from black lung disease, the argument being that they have exposed themselves to substantial health risks to satisfy the public interest in having cheap energy. Third, if a reasonable social objective is to use our health care system to save as many high quality life-years as possible within a limited health budget, and if it is correct that this is an objective that proponents of utilitarian or Rawlsian contractarian or radically egalitarian conceptions of justice could all endorse, then my judgment is that none of the proponents of these competing conceptions of justice would see totally implantable artificial hearts as a morally obligatory means to that end because there were too many alternative medical therapies that could save more life-years (with equal moral claim) at a lower cost.

We can complete our moral analysis on this point by turning around our original question and asking, would there be anything unjust about continuing funding for totally implantable artificial hearts until they are successfully developed? Here I would argue that a strong case can be made for saying that this would be unjust, not intrinsically, not in some possible health care systems in some very wealthy societies, but in the actual society that we find ourselves in today with the actual health policies we have in place for financing and distributing access to health care. Two contingent facts need to be noted here. First, the total cost of implanting a totally implantable artificial heart would be in the vicinity of $100,000 to $150,000 (in 1990 dollars). Second, unlike natural heart transplants, for which there are something like natural limits on the number that can be done (because it is related to the number of brain-dead head injury victims), there is no natural limit to the number of artificial hearts that might be produced. That limit would be determined by ability to pay. These are not the kinds of costs that most people could pay out of pocket, so it is reasonable to believe that the middle class would seek insurance protection through their employer-provided health benefit packages. This would drive up substantially the total cost of health care in our society, adding at least $30 billion per year to those costs. Both the middle class and businesses would try to find ways to reduce the burden of health costs to themselves, which they would do by squeezing funding for state Medicaid programs, which would mean that the poor would have less access to less adequate health care, and by squeezing hospitals for discounts, which would mean that hospitals could not engage in traditional practices of cost shifting so that they could provide uncompensated care to the uninsured working poor, whose access to care and quality of care would then be greatly compromised. (No one who reads this should think this is some fanciful philosophical scenario. This is essentially what is currently happening in our health care system.)[8]

Finally, if there are increased costs for health benefits for the middle class, then this means increased tax subsidies for the middle class as well, and those subsidies will be financed in part by the working poor, who will themselves be without health insurance and without access to totally implantable artificial hearts. In conclusion, if all this is true or very nearly true, then it seems any reasonable person would conclude that such an outcome is unjust; and if the dissemination of the totally implantable artificial heart would cause this to happen, then that would be an unjust technology to disseminate. Even a proponent of a libertarian conception of justice would see this total state of affairs as being unjust. Certainly neither the working poor nor the very poor would autonomously ratify as fair or just the dissemination of the artificial heart in these circumstances.

JUST GENETICS: THE CASE AGAINST GENETIC ENHANCEMENT TECHNOLOGIES

We can now return to our original problem: should we think of emerging genetic technologies as being on a moral par with all manner of other expensive life-saving medical technologies? That is, social beneficence might be understood as warranting social investment in the development and dissemination of these technologies but without considerations of justice that would *require* this. Alternatively, there are a large number of life-prolonging medical technologies that are competing for limited health resources, and society is free to use whatever criteria (moral or nonmoral) that seem reasonable, which is to say that emerging genetic technologies have no moral priority in this competition because they have no special moral status. As noted earlier, I will argue that considerations of justice do have relevance in this case and would warrant giving priority to some of these emerging genetic technologies. Specifically, I will argue that germ-line genetic engineering aimed at eliminating deleterious genes and replacing them with their properly functioning version would have such priority. By way of contrast, I will also argue that genetic engineering aimed at enhancing the genetic structure of an embryo makes no just claim on health resources, partially for reasons analogous to those that would disallow development of the artificial heart and partially for reasons that are peculiar to the domain of genetic justice.

I have in mind the following scenario: we have successfully developed germ-line genetic engineering. That is, we can take a four-cell embryo, place it under a very powerful scanning device hooked to a very powerful computer that analyzes its genetic structure, and identify those genes that are most likely to have serious deleterious effects on its future health, if it were allowed to develop and be born. If its genetic structure is very badly flawed, then it is simply discarded. But if it has ten or twenty genes that can be replaced, then this is done quickly and efficiently through the genetic engineering mechanisms that are available.

If we wish, we can imagine two scenarios here. In scenario "A," we are very proficient in using the technology, but the cost in 1990 dollars is still about $10,000 per engineered embryo. If every birth in the United States were so engineered, then the cost would be about $30 billion per year since there are roughly three million children born each year here. In scenario "B," we can imagine that we are not quite so proficient and the cost per engineered embryo is closer to $100,000. If every birth in America were to be engineered in that more costly scenario, then total costs would be about $300 billion per year, which is about forty-five percent of 1990 total health expenditures in the United States.

Before going on, I would like to dispense with some anticipated reader nitpicking. First, some might object that I have offered a fanciful philosopher's scenario from which we can learn nothing useful or reliable from a moral standpoint. In response, I would be prepared to argue that this is more a futuristic than a fanciful scenario. The seminal technology is in place that suggests that what I have described is a real world possibility.[9] Second, someone might argue that there is no perfectly perspicuous way to identify "deleterious" genes. I am operating with an admittedly very simpleminded and reductivist understanding of genes, failing to take into account the complex ways in which genetic heritage interacts with widely variable natural and social environmental factors. This is a reasonable criticism, and hence, I stipulate that "deleterious genes" will refer here to those genes that virtually all reasonable individuals would judge consistently to cause very premature death or serious health problems that drastically compromise the capacity of an individual to carry out virtually any near-normal life plan. Paradigm examples of the sort of genes I have in mind would be those for Huntington's disease, cystic fibrosis, or Tay–Sachs disease. Examples of the sort of genes I *do not* have in mind are those that might predispose an individual to coronary artery disease in the later stages of life. What I assume with respect to this latter example is that a predisposition is not a rigid determination, that individuals who knew themselves to be so disposed could modify their diet and lifestyle so as to minimize the actual risk of serious disease.

Third, I need to stress that for now I am talking about genetic engineering with respect to deleterious genes, as opposed to genetic engineering that would enhance genetically determined traits so that they might be expressed in a superior way rather than an average way, such as might be the case with memory skills. I will concede that there is an area of conceptual mushiness here, that sometimes a genetic modification can be described in either positive or negative terms, and that we may not have noncontroversial reasons for preferring one description rather than another. Still, there are many other circumstances in which it will be clear that we are talking about genetic enhancement.

I now wish to turn to a discussion of moral issues connected with genetic enhancement. My moral judgment in this regard is that it is much less likely that considerations of justice would require the development or dissemination of genetically enhancing technologies than technologies aimed at eliminating deleterious genes. Such genetically enhancing technologies are morally analogous to the development of totally implantable artificial hearts. Of course, someone might point out that if we are capable of eliminating deleterious genes and replacing them with their intact version, then it would require no radical technological innovation to replace a normal gene with a superior version of that gene. If this were true, then we would be faced with some serious and difficult problems of justice. The precise nature of these problems would depend upon the policies and practices in place for the financing and delivery of health care in our society. Let us consider two broad scenarios.

First, if this technology were paid for through private health insurance provided by employers and a train of consequences followed similar to those previously described for the artificial heart, then the same moral conclusion would follow, namely, that the uninsured working poor and the very poor on Medicaid would have been treated unjustly because the lot of those already well off had been improved at the expense of those who were already substantially less well off.

Second, we could imagine that we had in place a system of national health insurance, say, a very comprehensive system such as exists in Canada in which all individuals had essentially the same package of health benefits. Then the question would be whether to include genetic enhancement engineering as part of that package. Depending upon the cost of that technology, it would displace other possible therapeutic interventions, some of which might have a stronger claim to inclusion in that package from the perspective of justice. If it were excluded from the package, then the issue would be whether there was anything unjust about permitting those with sufficient resources to purchase the technology for their future progeny.

At first glance, it might seem that this would be no more morally problematic than sending one's children to elite private universities, the result being enhanced life opportunities to which less affluent parents would not have access for their children. But on more careful inspection there are more serious difficulties from the perspective of justice. After all, at least some children from economically impoverished circumstances who are intellectually gifted and highly motivated are given scholarships that permit them to attend elite universities and reap enhanced opportunities and rewards. This is what allows us as a society to pat ourselves on the back morally as committed to fair equality of opportunity. However, in the case of privately purchased genetic enhancement technology, there are no equivalent structures of fair equality of opportunity. That is, no four-cell embryo has the opportunity to merit access to that technology. Rather, the actual dissemination of the technology is determined strictly by willingness and ability to pay. There are, of course, many goods in our society that are distributed in this way. However, we have to recall that we are talking about germ-line genetic engineering. If the technology really does enhance native abilities substantially and effectively, contributing greatly to an enhanced sense of self-esteem, then that expands greatly *and fundamentally* the range of opportunities that will be available to that individual and presumably *to the descendants of that individual.* This would create the very definite possibility of a genetically permanent "master class." And even if we imagined this as a benign, nonoppressive master class, as Attanasio seems to have in mind,[10] this would still represent a prima facie unjust state of affairs because fair equality of opportunity would have been so significantly compromised.

There is one final moral conundrum that needs to be mentioned under the national health insurance scenario for genetic enhancement technology. On the assumption that we would not want to be unjust in our genetic enhancement decisions, what moral landmarks would we use for assuring ourselves that we were being fair enough in our genetic enhancement decisions? Again, I remind the reader that we are talking about four-cell embryos. As Agich[11] and DeNicola[12] point out, the normal moral reference points we use in connection with justice are entirely absent.

Does one four-cell embryo have any more of a just claim to an enhanced genetic endowment because of merit or desert or effort or productivity than any other? What about desire or respect for individual autonomy? This latter question has no obvious meaning in connection with a four-cell embryo, so we could hardly fail to treat this embryo justly if this is our moral reference point. The parents might well have strong preferences for such genetic enhancement, but it is not obvious that such preferences are sufficient to generate just claims for this technology.

Another common reference point for assessing just claims is need. Need as a moral reference point does have some applicability for our discussion in connection with deleterious genetic traits, although the connection is more indirect than direct. That is, the concept of need in health care requires some moral discipline so that needs are not just arbitrarily asserted. Callahan has observed, for example, that we tend to identify medical needs in our society in terms of whatever is at the edge of medical innovation, which procedure is useless for purposes of asserting the justness of competing claims.[13] By way of contrast, I think Daniels has got it right for the most part when he links needs that have a just claim to health resources with the degree to which fulfillment of such needs allows an individual to access a normal opportunity range in that society.[14] Thus, there are obvious ways in which cystic fibrosis or Tay–Sachs disease or a very large number of other genetic disorders effectively block an individual's access to that normal opportunity range. To return to our discussion, however, we are talking about genetic *enhancement* technologies, the kind of genetic interventions that might give an individual access to a superior opportunity range. Individuals may *want* to access that superior opportunity range, but they do not *need* to access that range, in the sense of need that would generate claims of justice.

Next, we might appeal to the concept of rights. I do not believe that a four-cell embryo has any rights at all, much less a right to an enhanced genetic endowment. But for the sake of argument and analysis, I will assume that such a right is a possibility, that it is a claim right and that it is rooted in some alleged interest that the embryo has in having an optimal range of life opportunities made available. If such a right exists, then we would have to specify somewhat precisely what that right gives an embryo a just claim to. That is, we would have to have some way of knowing when that claim right had been satisfied. However, if we try to think this through, we will quickly find ourselves in a complete conceptual muddle because there is no obvious natural limit to what might count as adequate genetic enhancement. Moreover, we are not just talking about some single genetic trait. We could conceivably be talking about thousands of genetic traits.

I would further remind the reader that this thought experiment is occurring in the context of a Canadian-style national health insurance plan, which is to say that we would have to be concerned about fair treatment of all citizens in this society, or at least all four-cell embryos that are going to be born. Presumably, all those embryos would start out as very genetically diverse. If we were to protect that diversity, and there are very good biological, social, and moral reasons for wanting to do that, then how would we know what counted as "fair genetic enhancement" of these embryos relative to one another? There would be enormous diversity and, hence, incomparability in this regard. How would we know whether we had done too much or too little in the way of genetic enhancement with respect to any given individual embryo? Life was a lot simpler when there was only the natural lottery, when all of us simply had to accept the fate that God or nature had imposed upon us. But if each and every genetic endowment is a product of human choice, then it seems we have an inescapable (but impossible) responsibility to make those choices as fairly as possible.

One further consideration is worthy of note: who exactly is the "we" that is supposed to have responsibility for making these choices for genetic enhancement? Is it some panel of experts who would have the moral right to shape in an absolutely fundamental and intimate way the lives of each and every future child, quite apart from the desires, preferences, and values of the parents of that child? That might be one way of ensuring a high degree of impartiality, but a high price would be paid in terms of other social values. Alternatively, we could allow parents to make their own genetic enhancement choices, although this would predictably yield substantial inequalities among those future children. Would the natural lottery be morally preferable from the perspective of justice, or at least the natural lottery stripped for the most part of deleterious genes? We turn now to answering that question.

JUST GENETICS: THE CASE FOR NEGATIVE GENETIC ENGINEERING

What are the considerations of justice that would warrant giving moral priority to genetic technologies that would eliminate deleterious genes over other kinds of emerging life-saving or life-enhancing medical technologies? To begin answering this question, we must appeal to some conception of justice that would command widespread rational assent. As we noted earlier, and as Agich and De-Nicola have argued, traditional theories of justice have nothing useful to offer in this regard, the primary reason being that these theories all operate in a world in which natural assets and liabilities are assumed as given. But with the emergence of genetic technologies, that assumption is justifiably called into question. Again, what both Agich and DeNicola argue is that a Rawlsian contractarian conception of justice is the only conception of justice that gives us a handle for determining what might count as a just distribution of genetic resources.[15] The virtue of Rawls' position is that he offers a fair procedure for determining distributions, which involves assuming the original position behind a veil of ignorance. Although Rawls himself has very little to say about genetic choices (because this was a barely imaginable option at the time he wrote *A Theory of Justice,* roughly 1970), and although his theory of justice tolerates a broad range of inequalities in our social life and he is inclined to think that we ought to remedy natural inequalities through choosing appropriate social policies and practices, it is relatively easy to make a case for saying that Rawls would support the genetically engineered elimination of deleterious genes as something required by justice. One obvious reason for saying this is that there are numerous genetic disorders that cause very premature death or profound disabilities that virtually exclude that individual from effective participation in any portion of our society, and that *no amount of remedial social policy or more just social practices will effectively correct for those losses.* The only effective corrective is the genetic engineering we described. Further, one of the substantive moral reference points for Rawls is the plight of those who are least well off. Changes in social policy are just only to the extent that they improve the lot of the least well off. Certainly those who are afflicted with the very serious genetic disorders that we have in mind have a legitimate claim to be considered among those who are least well off so far as health care justice is concerned.

A critic might respond that there are alternatives, such as gene therapy, that are less radical than genetic engineering. However, as I hinted earlier, gene therapy might not generate just claims in the way that genetic engineering would. This is not a moral judgment that I can make with absolute confidence because the actual facts, such as they might prove to be in the future, can make a large difference. Right now gene therapy is more like a half-way technology that temporarily corrects a medical deficiency, but does not actually cure the disorder. If this were to remain true for the indefinite future, then gene therapy would have to compete on the same moral plane as a host of other half-way life-prolonging medical technologies, such as organ transplants and dialysis. That is, gene therapy would have no intrinsic claim to moral priority over any of these other technologies. And even if it were a very successful technology, the moral question would still need to be raised: why would we prefer this to germ-line genetic engineering, especially if we could be reasonably confident that germ-line engineering would delete the defective gene from all succeeding generations?[16]

There is an obvious answer to our last question, namely, that germ-line genetic engineering is not a therapeutic option for someone who is already born. For that individual, the only choices are gene therapy, however imperfect it may be as a therapy, or passive acceptance of one's genetic fate, which might be very gruesome. Of course, if a society had sufficient resources to completely fund both unlimited gene therapy and our genetic engineering program, then we would have bought our way out of that moral dilemma. That, however, is a fanciful scenario. There are limits to what any society can spend to meet competing, virtually unlimited health needs.

If we imagine that some sort of choice must be made between funding a very large potential demand for gene therapy, say, $30 billion per year, and funding my genetic engineering program at the $30 billion level, and if we have only $35 billion to spend on these health needs, then what would count as a just allocation of these resources? This has all the appearances of a terrible and irresolvable problem of intergenerational conflict.

Daniels has one approach for dealing with what appear to be problems of intergenerational conflict, and that is to transform them into problems of allocating health resources over the course of one's own life. He uses this approach to achieve a creative solution to the problem of what counts as a just allocation of health resources to the elderly.[17] This approach has considerable rational appeal with regard to our current problem since it seems that it would be eminently prudent to eliminate from the very beginning of my life those deleterious genetic predispositions that are most likely to compromise seriously the length and/or quality of my life later. However, the reason why Daniels' original strategy is so creative and feasible is that the current generation of the young and middle-aged are making rationing decisions for their *future* selves that contribute to the enhancement of their own current life prospects. But in the situation we are faced with, the current generation in need of gene therapy would simply be shifting resources to another generation, if they were to relinquish their claims to those resources.

At this point we might invoke Rawls' original position—the veil of ignorance argument, or a variation thereof. That is, assume that we are all noumenal selves who know nothing unique about ourselves, that we know that at some point in our social history we will invent the genetic technology I described earlier, and that we do not know which generation it is that we belong to so that, for example, we might belong to the generation that needs (and can only use) gene therapy or we might belong to the generation that would benefit near conception from genetic engineering. Under these assumptions, what principles of justice would we appeal to for purposes of determining a fair distribution? I assume my readers are familiar with Rawls' principles of justice, which I do not see as offering that much by way of resolving this particular moral dispute. As noted earlier, one standard reference point is the plight of those who are least well off. That is precisely what is up for grabs in this dispute since, if one side or the other receives the bulk of these resources, the result will be that the other side will be able to claim that they are now among those who are least well off in terms of health.

At this point we can invoke Daniels' original strategy in thinking about problems of health care justice. That is, Daniels devises a version of Rawls' fair equality of opportunity principle which he then uses to determine what counts as a more or less fair distribution of health resources in our society. The general idea is that health resources ought to be distributed so that all have an opportunity to access a normal opportunity range in that society, that is, the range of life plans that are available in that society.[18] It is this moral perspective that gives considerable moral weight to the genetic engineering approach we have described in competition for limited health resources. Eliminating deleterious genes, more than anything else offered by medical science, would seem to ensure fair access to a normal opportunity range for individuals who would otherwise be extremely deprived in the distribution of societal benefits. With this in mind, we move back behind Rawls' veil of ignorance.

We have individuals who have a sense of justice, who do not know which generation it is they belong to, and whose sense of health care justice requires that they distribute health resources so that they maximize the likelihood that each individual will have a fair opportunity to access a normal opportunity range. What follows from that? We might imagine someone saying that it is unfortunate that the current generation is not able to benefit from germ-line genetic engineering, but that is not unjust since this was simply an outcome of the natural lottery over which no one could exercise much control. By way of contrast, if the current generation were to deny this future generation access to germ-line corrective genetic therapy, then that would be unjust. Therefore, this future generation has a just claim to the $30 billion needed to ensure this future generation an intact genetic structure.

But then we have to remember that an integral part of Rawls' contractarian perspective is the hypothetical assent that all parties to the social contract give to the principles of justice that will govern that society, which I am extending to include the more specific principles of health care justice. I do not believe that I have that assent from the current generation to the proposed distribution. I suspect that they would have a justified claim that they were treated unjustly if this last proposal were insisted upon. To rectify this, we have to imagine some sort of exchange of benefits between these generations. What we need to equalize is fair equality of opportunity for the members of both generations, which would include comparable exposure to the risk of premature death. Daniels' life span account does offer some helpful moral clues at this point. What we need to imagine is that this future generation, which will reap very large ensured health benefits from germ-line genetic engineering, would be willing to give up access to some very expensive life-prolonging medical interventions at later stages of life, by which I mean stages of life as early as middle age. After all, they have been granted, virtually from conception, protection against a very large number of life-threatening and life-diminishing genetic disorders. The willingness of this future generation to give up access to some of these future medical technologies, which some members of that generation will most certainly need because they will still be susceptible to a host of medical problems that are not genetically determined, will free up resources that the current generation can use to purchase gene therapy for its members up to that point at which the members of both generations will have roughly comparable opportunity ranges and ranges of risk for premature death. That is, individual members of each generation will end up dying prematurely or having something less than access to a normal opportunity range, but they will not be able to claim that they have been treated unfairly because this will once again be a product of the natural lottery (and a social agreement between the generations). This would strike me as a plausible and fair outcome, not to mention its being a feasible bargain between the generations. But this is not an outcome that would simply be dictated by principles of justice derived from either Rawls or Daniels. Rather, this reflects a constructivistic approach sensitive to the moral contours of genetic justice.

CONCLUSIONS

In summary, I have argued that there are unique moral contours to the problems of justice that will be posed by emerging genetic technologies. That is, whatever principles of justice yield morally defensible results with respect to the distribution of, say, transplantable hearts or access to scarce ICU beds, will not yield similarly defensible results through some straightforward application of these principles to emerging genetic technologies. This is in part because these technologies undercut one of the bedrock factual assumptions on which our usual conceptions of justice rest, namely, that our genetic heritage (and the burdens and opportunities it might represent) is a given.

I have also tried to illustrate what some of those contours of genetic justice might look like. In particular, I noted that genetic engineering aimed at eliminating deleterious genes has a strong claim from the perspective of health care justice for research funds that would lead to its successful development and dissemination. More precisely, this is a moral claim that is much stronger than the claims of virtually all the very expensive half-way life-prolonging technologies that have been the hallmark of late twentieth century medicine, including gene therapy. We hasten to add, however, that this is a conclusion that holds true only within the context of a system of comprehensive national health insurance, such as exists in Canada. In the actual system of health care financing currently prevailing in the United States, the likelihood is that advances in genetic engineering will only add to the substantial injustices that already characterize our health care system since it is likely that the middle class and well off will benefit disproportionately from these advances to the detriment of those who are least well off, and will now be made even worse off. Genetic engineering aimed at eliminating deleterious genes from the gene pool has considerable moral promise for protecting fair equality of opportunity in our society, but only if it is in fact available to all in our society who otherwise would be afflicted with these deleterious genes.

One final observation is worth making. We like to believe that liberalism and justice are inseparable moral ideals. But there will be problems in maintaining our commitment to both these ideals. For example, if we did perfect the techniques of negative genetic engineering so that we could eliminate from four-cell embryos most of the more devastating genetically based disorders with which we are familiar, then could a just and liberal society require, as a matter of public policy, that *all* conceptions occur *in vitro* so that this engineering could be done for the benefit of that future person, even over the objections of religious individuals who saw this as secular humanism run amok? It would take another paper simply to begin to sort out the relevant moral issues. But these issues are there. They are very much part of the unique contours of genetic justice.

NOTES

1. Munson and Davis have in fact argued that there is a strong social obligation requiring the development of these technologies. See Ronald Munson and Lawrence Davis, "Germ-Line Gene Therapy and the Medical Imperative," *Kennedy Institute of Ethics Journal* 2 (1992): 137–58.

2. Michael Walzer, *Spheres of Justice: A Defense of Pluralism and Equality* (New York: Basic Books, 1983), especially chap. 1.

3. Leonard M. Fleck, "Just Health Care (I): Is Beneficence Enough?" *Theoretical Medicine* 10 (1989): 167–182; and "Just Health Care (II): Is Equality Too Much?" *Theoretical Medicine* 10 (1989): 301–310.

4. John Rawls, "Kantian Constructivism in Moral Theory," *The Journal of Philosophy* 72 (1980): 515–572.

5. John Rawls, "Justice as Fairness: Political Not Metaphysical," *Philosophy and Public Affairs* 14 (1985): 223–251.

6. Leonard M. Fleck, "DRGs: Justice and the Invisible Rationing of Health Care Resources," *The Journal of Medicine and Philosophy* 12 (1987): 165–196, especially pp. 165–176 which offers a detailed outline of the framework of nonideal justice. For another application of this framework to Oregon's approach to health care rationing, see Fleck's essay, "The Oregon Medicaid Experiment: Is It Just Enough?" *Business and Professional Ethics Journal* 9 (1990): 201–217.

7. William Schwartz, "The Inevitable Failure of Current Cost Containment Strategies," *The Journal of the American Medical Association* 257 (1987): 220–224.

8. Helen Burstin, Stuart Lipsitz, and Troyen Brennan, "Socioeconomic Status and Risk for Substandard Medical Care," *Journal of the American Medical Association* 268 (1992): 2383–2387.

9. See Yury Verlinsky, Eugene Pargament, and Charles Strom, "The Preimplantation Genetic Diagnosis of Genetic Diseases," *Journal of In-Vitro Fertilization and Embryo Transfer* 7 (1990): 1–5; A. Dokras et al., "Trophectoderm

Biopsy in Human Blastocysts," *Human Reproduction,* 5 (1990): 821–825. More generally, see Andrea Bonnicksen, "Genetic Diagnosis of Human Embryos," *The Hastings Center Report* 22 (1992, suppl.): S5–S11.

10. John B. Attanasio, "The Constitutionality of Regulating Human Genetic Engineering: Where Procreative Liberty and Equal Opportunity Collide," *The University of Chicago Law Review* 53 (1986): 1274–1342.

11. George Agich, "Genetic Justice," *University of Western Ontario Law Review* 24 (1986): 39–50.

12. Daniel R. DeNicola, "Genetics, Justice, and Respect for Human Life," *Zygon* 11 (1976): 115–137.

13. Daniel Callahan, *What Kind of Life: The Limits of Medical Progress* (New York: Simon and Schuster, 1990), 31–68.

14. Norman Daniels, *Just Health Care* (Cambridge, U.K.: Cambridge University Press, 1985), 36–58.

15. Agich, "Genetic Justice," 47–50; DeNicola, "Genetics, Justice, and Respect," 116–124.

16. We concede that there is always the possibility of future genetic mutations, but an effective technique for genetic engineering would at least offer reasonable hope that *this* genetic deficiency would not turn up again in this family line.

17. Norman Daniels, *Am I My Parents' Keeper: An Essay on Justice Between the Young and the Old* (Oxford, U.K.: Oxford University Press, 1988), 66–82.

18. Daniels, *Just Health Care,* 36–48.

9
JUSTICE AND THE LIMITATIONS OF GENETIC KNOWLEDGE

Marc A. Lappé

In the next decade, the human genome project will come of age, as about 100,000 different human genes and their supporting infrastructure yield to molecular inquiry. Previous commentators on the ethical issues raised by this project have often centered their analysis on the proprietary uses of genetic knowledge, confidentiality, and the requirements for protection of individuals against potential discrimination.[1] This essay will focus on the implications of the project for the treatment of human differences under certain social policies and programs.

Early in the decoding of the human genome, researchers believed that genetic data would be useful primarily in a medical context. The National Center for Human Genome Research, for example, has stated that genetic information "... will provide new strategies to diagnose, treat, and possibly prevent human diseases."[2] While this objective was a major selling point for the genome project in the late 1980s, it is clear that benefits of this kind represent only a portion of the true scope of the genome program.

Even as recently as 1992, the genome project continued to be described in limited terms. For instance, the brochure used in the early 1990s by the U.S. Department of Health and Human Services to summarize the project limited its significance to medical developments and two additional areas: (1) understanding the process of embry-

onic development and, (2) uncovering genomic sequences that reveal human ancestry.[3]

Despite the addition of these latter elements, this description still
provides only an incomplete and modest depiction of what will be
accessible once the human genome is fully described. The scope of
genetic data that will be gleaned from the genome project is almost
certain to eclipse simple descriptions of single-gene associated disease, mutations that disrupt embryogenesis, or genetic markers that
help us trace our ancestry. At a minimum, it is evident that genomic
researchers will uncover much of the data needed to decipher the
molecular code for functional genes that directly and indirectly affect the timing, sequence, and operation of specific organs. Researchers will continue to uncover the blocks of genes analogous to the
"homeobox" genes in fruit flies and mice which govern embryologic
development. In so doing, they will gain more than a simple understanding of embryogenesis: developmental phenomena and embryonic defects will be subject to a new degree of biomedical analysis
and control. With preimplantation diagnosis, preferential implantation of HOX-gene "normal" embryos may become the norm, opening the door to a new form of micro-eugenics.

Most critically, the genome project teams will unveil data about
the genetic *predisposition to* (not merely the *occurrence of*) disease. This
is especially significant from the perspective of the distribution of
societal resources (e.g., from a national health insurance pool) because it is likely that substantial gene-based differences in human
proclivities to infectious organisms or environmental agents will be
revealed in advance of actual disease. Such uncovery of disease pred-
ilection has already received much attention and concern, as shown
by the papers in this volume that deal with insurance and genetic
screening.

As new gene sequences are revealed, it is most likely that they will
be cross-correlated with detailed interactive maps of all other genetic
loci in the genome. This interpretation will involve complex integra-
tive technology to compare and interpret genome sequences at great
chromosomal distances from one another. With this capacity, a much
more complex picture of gene action and its significance for human
traits will probably become accessible. Most compellingly, polygenic
traits (those associated with multiple genetic loci and environmental
factors, acting in concert) will become amenable to a level of analy-

sis heretofore not possible with standard linkage and heritability analyses.

This means that we will learn more about why individuals as well as groups differ from one another in diseases such as hypertension, heart disease, and cancer. Indeed, it is this very issue of group profiling that raises important questions of equity for social policy in the areas of discrimination and compensation.

GROUP VERSUS INDIVIDUAL DIFFERENCES

Even as the genetic language has proven to be universal, we have learned that the content of each person's genetic makeup is different. This uniqueness provides a basis for differentiating biological individuality and provides the starting point for a whole new field of forensic genotyping. Currently this fine genetic differentiation is considered relevant for issues such as paternity testing, criminal identification, and tissue grafting in which precise gene-based matches are critical.[4] In a medical context, individual genetic profiles have proven useful primarily for identifying those families whose members express deviant genotypes sufficient to cause clinically relevant disease so that more precise counseling and/or prenatal diagnosis can be offered. The question of how much of these data are relevant to public health has yet to be addressed fully.

A key question in this regard is to what extent if any, the genome project will reveal *group* differences in the frequency of major genetic loci that affect signficant human attributes. To date, this possibility has been given short shrift primarily because of the presumption that genetic material is widely distributed and rarely unique. Indeed, much of the focus on the genome has stressed its presumptive universality or extensive commonality. Emphasizing that *only* two to ten million nucleotide bases (out of three billion) differ from person to person, Mark Guyer of the National Center for Human Genetic Research (NCHGR) has stated that "most of the information in that map will pertain to everyone."[5]

As shown by the spate of recent correspondence in *Science* pertaining to the overlap or lack thereof of unique genetic identifiers in forensic work, scientists are still uncertain whether some genetic data will prove to be unique to certain groups or if some data may not be found in all people of even closely related groups.[6] Marked genetic variance has been found for some rare blood group polymorphisms,[7] alpha-1-antitrypsin alleles,[8] and other complex loci where certain groups (e.g., the Lapps, Eskimos, and certain African tribal peoples) have genes that are exclusive to their common ancestry.

The commonly held view that genetic mutations will always generate a few aberrant genes in unrelated groups (as has proven true for the genes that determine Tay–Sachs disease among non-Ashkenazi Jews), and that subsequent genetic "churning" will ensure the eventual intermixing of these genes with the gene pool as a whole, may not hold up over time. Rare genotypes are rare because of their genetic isolation and are commonly found among groups separated by long evolutionary intervals. Heterozygote selection may increase the frequency of such genes (as is the case for the hemoglobinopathies), and Hardy–Weinberg equilibria may describe their new incidence figures in interbreeding populations. But, as Lewontin and Hartl emphasize, such equilibria are of little value for detecting variation among subgroups—and major genetic differences are likely to exist among historically isolated populations.[9]

By analogy to human cancer incidence data, which reveal major group-specific differences in site-specific cancer rates, some major genetically based characteristics may be found to differ systematically from group to group. There already may be such a prominent example in the gene products determined by the *Lp(a)* locus. Humans can have levels of *Lp(a)* that vary over a thousand-fold range, with most people having very low levels. Those who have high levels are at increased risk of heart disease. However, this risk is currently limited to those of Caucasian ancestry. Those of African ancestry appear to have other risk factors that are more important for determining cardiovascular status.

The level of this lipoprotein, which is associated with either a "healthy" phenotype (little heart disease) or "high risk" phenotype (much heart disease), is determined by the number of copies of certain sequences in this gene. People with smaller than average numbers of these duplicate regions have high *Lp(a)* levels and are much more likely to have heart disease than are those with multiple sequence copies whose *Lp(a)* levels are lower. About thirty percent of patients whose heart disease began at an early age will have *Lp(a)* levels above those of the general population norms. This protein may be involved in promoting the formation of blood clots or arteriosclerotic lesions that eventually clog the heart's arteries. Most interestingly, it appears to be an independent risk factor from those traditionally linked to heart disease, such as cholesterol levels or blood pressure.

Because *Lp(a)* also predicts the severity of heart disease, it is almost certainly going to be a candidate for clinical testing and perhaps for preenrollment screening for insurers as well. While the blood level of this factor cannot yet be predictably influenced by drugs or dietary regimen, it is particularly important to consider what might be gained by instituting early screening. At least one prominent human geneticist has suggested that we may wish to institute intensive environmental measures to modify *Lp(a)* levels once we have uncovered the increased risk status linked to the gene.[10]

But since only the risk status of whites is presently tied to this gene, instituting screening and follow-up testing and prophylaxis (should that become available) to the rest of the population is problematic. Will people of African-American ancestry or Hispanics benefit or be harmed by such a policy were they not to be screened? Excluding groups from presumptive prophylactic measures is potentially discriminatory. This is because African-Americans who are at the same or higher risk of cardiovascular disease may be better identified by other, as yet unascertained, loci and correspondingly benefitted by alternative risk reduction measures. Instituting a genetic screening program that focused solely on *Lp(a)* alleles could mean that minority populations would receive fewer health benefits simply because another "white" genetic locus had been described before the comparable genes had been identified in another risk group. Of course, should adverse effects stem from such screening (e.g., employment discrimination) then African-Americans may in fact be better off if their competitiveness for employment is increased by the screening of other populations.

The counterargument that complete knowledge of the human genome will fill in all data gaps and eventually result in equity for all groups fails to be convincing because it assumes that the risk profiles of groups—in terms of health risks and economic and social access—will all balance out once the full genomic complement of each group is ascertained. That is, the social costs of adverse health outcomes among such groups as African-Americans which have certain predispositions (presumably genetically based) to illnesses such as hypertension will be counterbalanced by the differential health risks carried by having a predominantly Caucasian genetic background. Such an eventuality is extremely unlikely given the extent of genetic divergence among groups resulting from disparate selection pressures on populations that have historically had predominantly urban versus rural life styles. Were substantial ethnic-based group differences to be found in the distribution of major disease-associated genetic loci, the fact that access to health is unequal among many such groups has clear ethical implications. This is especially true in a society such as that of the United States which has not yet adopted any version of universal health insurance. (See, e.g., the essays in this volume by Robert J. Pokorski and Norman Daniels.)

SIGNIFICANCE OF GROUP DIFFERENCES

Certain gene-associated human characteristics other than health factors may also differ among groups. Such behavioral characteristics having significant social utility or disutility—tendencies toward altruism or violence, predisposition to mental illness, mental acuity or intelligence, and maternal instinct—would require considerable rethinking if shown to be associated with a group-specific genomic profile. The traditional view is that these factors are highly conditioned and shaped by social and other environmental forces, and hence to speak about genetic determination of any measured group differences (e.g., in intelligent quotients) as being largely or wholly "genetic" in origin is erroneous.[11] But on the basis of animal models from behavioral genetics, many behavioral characteristics have been shown to be polygenic and will prove to have a strong genetic component. These group associations would be made even more problematic if they were also divided along socioeconomic lines.

Certain key conditions already show social gradients in their incidence. For instance, many psychiatric disorders as well as major diseases such as cancer, heart disease, and hypertension are distributed along a steep socioeconomic gradient. Poor people and those with less education commonly experience a higher incidence of many diseases in these categories than do their well-to-do, better educated brethren. Because in the United States, poverty is frequently linked to ethnicity, and ethnicity in turn reflects major differences in certain gene frequencies, attempts to identify genetic components of these

trends has been inherently suspect as racist and a prejudicial aban-
donment of egalitarian values.

However, recent studies of emigres in Israel suggest that some of
the social (environmental) explanation for the high concentration
of disease among low socioeconomic classes may be only partially
correct. Researchers have now shown that while depression is closely
associated with environmental correlates of low social status (especially in women), the concentration of cases of schizophrenia among
people in low socioeconomic groups shows a strong pattern consistent with genetic selection.[12] In the researchers' view, this disorder—
and by inference, others that show a steep socioeconomic gradient—
can be the result of a social "sifting" of persons with genetic predisposition to poorer coping skills into the lowermost rungs of the social
order where their reproduction furthers the spread of the responsible genotypes.

CONSEQUENCES OF GENETIC INEQUALITY IN THE SOCIAL ORDER

The assumption that the human genetic proclivity for these and any
other valued or unvalued traits is unknowable, or that environmental
factors will always skew genetic causation, may not hold. First, it would
be imprudent to believe that complexity alone will thwart the accessibility of polygenic human traits to analysis. As we have seen, the
process of decoding the genome will almost certainly include a process of cross-correlation and integration of multiple loci as they interplay in shaping characteristics and features of the whole person.

We can be reasonably sure of discovering the genetic precondition
of a range of complex human traits by looking at the history of other
traits and disorders once thought to be intractable to reductionist
analysis. A case in point is depression, a psychological disorder once
thought to defy biochemical explication. As mentioned earlier, recent studies have shown that several forms of depression, including
the bipolar form of manic depressive illness, fit quite nicely into biochemical and genetic analysis.[13]

The increasing scope and explanatory power of the genome project generally, and population genetics specifically, means that many
of these most crucial human attributes—including the distribution
of illness, senescence, learning skills, and competence—may also fall

to genetic explanations, at least in part. This inference is drawn from parallel studies in animals, especially mice, which show that disease susceptibility, aging, and learning ability are all controlled to some degree by multiple genetic loci.[14] Such traits clearly involve a delicate and complex interplay between environmental and genetic factors. However, a strong likelihood exists that these genes are not randomly distributed among groups of individuals with disparate ancestry (ethnic origins). While the creators of the human genome project see such a likelihood as raising scientifically interesting questions about human origins, the existence of group-specific differences in key human attributes has more ominous overtones: it raises the specter of eugenic policies, discrimination, and oppression. This is particularly so in light of the history of misapplications of human genetics and social theory and the use of false science in shaping malevolent eugenic theory. What will be different after the genome project is that there will be substantial "hard" science pointing to group differences. What uses, if any, such data are put to for shaping social policy must be considered now.

IMPLICATIONS OF INEQUITABLE GENOMIC DISTRIBUTION

When and if a given genetic sequence proves instructive about such polygenic traits as intelligence, emotionality, or affective illness integrating these new facts into public policy will be fraught with moral and political difficulty. The tendency will be to ignore such data for all but medical purposes. At the simplest level, this is because the formulation of equitable policies presupposes a "veil of ignorance" behind which policy is made. First expounded by John Rawls, the ignorance principle holds that policies are best made under the assumption that anyone could be in a given reference group.[15] The effect of such a principle is to prevent groups from using social policy as an instrument of their own exclusive advantage. Because everyone must consider themselves to be potentially in the worst-off group, the tendency of policy formulations under a Rawlsian system of justice is to have people identify with and protect the interests of those who are most disadvantaged.

In large measure, the heuristic appeal of this approach turned on the reality (about 1971, when it was first proposed) that we could not know all of the salient features of people. Nor could we know in what way the natural lottery distributed poor lots to some and good lots to others. However, ignorance of salient differences cannot be an ingredient of "just" social policies when such differences not only exist but can in fact be known and identified. It is now clear that the curve of "normalcy" that underlies virtually all significant human traits is fractured and partitioned into several very discrete polygenic domains. Just as the bell-shaped curve of human height contains individuals with both pituitary dwarfism and gigantism, so will the bell-shaped curve of normalcy for the distribution of risks to heart disease be found to be bifurcated again and again into high and low risk groups.

How we handle this information is as much a moral question as a political one. How should we distribute societal goods (such as jobs) and support (such as universal health insurance) among high risk populations? Who should pay and how much should they pay for these benefits? Should we compensate or ignore costly gene-based predilections for disease or disability? It may prove possible to design policies that acknowledge certain gene-based proclivities toward illness as parts of programs that compensate for disability rather than penalize the holders of certain traits—whether those traits are socially valued or disvalued.

The extent, if any, to which we are obliged to recognize such human differences in terms of compensating those who are disadvantaged will be put to an acid test in the postgenome years. Will we consider ourselves to be duty bound to compensate for the distribution of genetic disadvantages while accepting an obligation to respect the distribution of genetic advantages? These questions require that we rethink the issues of justice, deservedness, and duties in a new light.

While many groups with genetic infirmities have attracted public empathy and support, it is not clear that the U.S. public is ready or willing to recognize group differences other than those that directly pertain to genetic susceptibility to illness. (Witness, for example, the racist overtones of the I.Q. and heredity debate). Answers to these questions may require a different approach to the philosophy of equity and justice. Genes for such traits as intellect are almost certainly going to be found to be inequitably distributed among groups of people as they are now known to be so distributed among individuals.

Existing ethical theories about differences and their adjudication usually assume that random events contribute to this so-called natural lottery. Once those events fall under conscious control, what comprises a "fair share" versus a "poor share" of the genetic lottery (say, for intellectual traits) will of necessity become a social problem. While overt efforts to control this lottery will almost certainly be resisted (for all the reasons that contemporary eugenic measures are opposed in this country), even the simple disclosure of genetic compositions will perforce reveal human differences that warrant some attention.

MORAL AND SOCIAL CHALLENGES OF THE GENOME PROJECT

The products of the genome project may throw into stark relief the paradox of a society based on the premise of equal standing at creation and one that is found to be composed of a genetically heterogeneous group of subpopulations with qualitatively different frequencies of heritable traits. As a society, we will have to ask if we can in fact collect information that reveals these individual differences and still continue to treat all individuals the same. We may wish to consider some people, by virtue of their gene-based handicaps or predispositions, to have greater (or lesser) claims on us for support (especially if that support is limited to job opportunity and health coverage). Others, by virtue of their inheritance of larger than normal genetic loads (because of their exposure to genotoxins or high inbreeding coefficients) may have claims on us for still other protection or compensation. And still others may be the genetic equivalents of the nonsmoking populations in terms of their projected fitness (in a non-Darwinian sense) and therefore have certain claims on us for recognition or compensation (e.g., special insurance rates).

What is clear is that even a partial picture of the genetic landscape that defines the molecular differences among human individuals will reveal more in its nonuniformity than in its hoped for universality. This landscape is likely to be one that is jagged and uneven, broken by genetic discontinuities among cultural and ethnic groups. Genes will not be partitioned either uniformly or fairly among groups with disparate genetic heritages. This means that by its nature, the genetic lottery will show itself to be manifestly unfair. But fairness is only a valid concept when outcomes or measures to achieve a certain end-point are under human control or dominion. We do not think that lightning strikes are "unfair," but we do think that poorly grounded cables that permit such strikes to injure people to be unfair. In a broad sense, a similar analogy applies to genetics.

Hence, the partitioning of the genetic lottery is not in and of itself manifestly unfair: genes are normally distributed by purely chance events of recombination and assortment. This is why the Hardy–Weinberg law applies universally. But once genetic loci are known that have mutational "hot spots" or when individuals are identifiable with particularly "risky" genotypes (e.g., those carrying the genes for Fanconi's anemia, xeroderma pigmentosum, ataxia telangietasia, or the newly discovered markers for breast cancer), the consequences of their reproductive activities for their own children and future generations become knowable and hence potentially controllable. Will we be able to resist the pressures to break from the past tradition of totally "neutral" genetic counseling in which nondirectiveness is the goal? Or will we feel compelled to recognize these differences as being salient and important for future generations?

Clearly, we will know with much greater precision what populations will have disproportionately high gene frequencies for certain deleterious traits or predispositions—at least as those traits are now measured against present environments. Some traits that had selective advantages in past environments will be recognized as part of the genetic load for contemporary environments. Other populations that have been isolated culturally and historically from the mainstream of human affairs will exist as genetic islands, with archaic and perhaps inappropriate genotypes for modern human environments. Many of these populations presently exist in rural developing countries. Such people will be unlikely to receive the same kind and degree of benefits from the genome project as will their more fortunate peers in developed countries, if for no other reason than that the diseases afflicting affluent populations include more disorders having genetic proclivities than do those of the rural poor.[16]

Some people in industrialized countries will be found to be unusually robust and tolerant of the stringent conditions common to the toxic environments characteristic of some worksites. For instance, people who can only metabolize certain chemicals slowly (so-called slow acetylators) are at higher risk for cancers (especially bladder cancer) than are their faster metabolizing co-workers.[17] A still unanswered major ethical dilemma is whether or not to use such information in genetic screening programs in potentially toxic work sites.[18] Social and political forces may ask that those who carry a disproportionate load in terms of genetic heritage carry a disproportionate, increased share of the responsibility and cost of health insurance, job training, and other benefits. Moral reasoning may reach the exact opposite conclusions. Those who are least well off may arguably be given certain social advantages to compensate for their otherwise unavoidable genetic infirmities, for instance, by putting them into a "high risk pool" of insurance applicants or by expanding the gambit of the present day acts to protect people with disabilities. But in doing so, we will also be expanding the penumbra of discrimination and social stigma to groups whose infirmities were once hidden and private matters.

CONCLUSIONS

We will need to garner much wisdom to know how to apply the data that we glean from the human genome project and how to ensure that it is used morally. Among the options that will become available at each phase of the genome project are the following:

1. accrue data and use it to establish prevalence figures for key human traits;
2. put data into banks that permit access to group information;
3. use data to identify and provide counseling to individuals at risk for perpetuating serious disorders;
4. use data to redress inequalities in apparant apportionment of genes that confer disadvantages to holders; and
5. use data to design eugenic strategies.

These independent alternatives are arrayed in ascending order of controversy. Simple acquisition of genetic data unlinked to individuals by name or address provides a basis for establishing gene frequencies and prevalence figures. But to be truly useful in any epidemiological sense, genetic data will also have to be associated or linked to people by virtue of their extended mating groups, geography, and health patterns. Here, issues of confidentiality must certainly come into play or problems of potential discrimination will inevitably occur.

Using genome data for counseling purposes, or for that matter, forensic work and genetic identification programs, is a logical extension of existing programs. While not without ethical problems, there are few novel issues drawn out by these applications. Using genetic data to design social programs that address the issues of inequalities is a major novel consideration. For instance, if it were shown that certain human leukocyte antigen (HLA) markers put individuals of particular ancestry at risk for autoimmune disorders, it might be appropriate to design strategies to pinpoint the carriers of the particular markers and alert them (and their caregivers) to the possibility of adverse reactions. A case in point is the genetic predisposition to silicosis and rheumatic disorders. While the responsible genetic locus is most prevalent among people of Japanese ancestry,[19] alerting people who are potential sandblasters or other workers to their risk status would be a justifiable use of these data. Use by employers to exclude such individuals from employment is a much more controversial application.

At the terminus of the application of these data are those in the general population who might be at increased risk for autoimmune disease. Such people would be potential candidates for counseling before they received breast implants or other interventions with the possibility of stimulating the immune system.

Use of genome data for eugenic purposes, whether tacitly or by policy, is the most controversial policy of all. In the past, the medical and public health communities have had to handle human differences in each extant generation as they arose and expressed themselves in predilections to disease and disability. But with advanced knowledge of the consequences of reproduction, it is inevitable that eugenic questions will be raised about supporting or not supporting certain group or individual decisions about procreation.

Even as these data become increasingly probative and reliable, it would be a great mistake to use such knowledge to compel, coerce, or otherwise discourage procreative decision making. The present policies that favor free reproductive choice are based on the premise of equal standing and deservedness of people with greatly dissimilar backgrounds and makeups. Genetic data may further refine such differences, but provide no real guidance as to the deservedness of any group of individuals for support or sanction for their procreative decisions. Different policies may prove appropriate for those who are the genetic equivalents of the nonsmoking population in terms of their projected fitness. For these people, accepting their genetic status as conferring better than normal odds of future well-being may mean nothing more than ensuring that policies are not adopted that penalize them for their good fortune. Benefits, in terms of tracking, rewards, or similar incentives, may not be appropriate since the genetic lottery has conferred its own reward.

We may wish to consider whether or not some people by virtue of their gene-based handicaps or predispositions have greater claims on us for support than do those whose genetic makeup is largely "normal." This is especially true if that support is limited to job opportunity where we have determined that handicaps of this kind should not reduce the employability of otherwise qualified applicants. We may also wish to consider the appropriateness of selective policies for those who carry larger than normal genetic loads by virtue of their nonconsensual workplace or environmental exposure to genotoxins or (less arguably) to socially induced high inbreeding coefficients. For these people, the choice to play the genetic lottery on a level playing field has been compromised by societal actions. Arguments of justice support the claim that many such genomically impaired people have claims on us for other forms of compensation just as did the Hiroshima women who came to the United States for plastic surgery after the war.

Knowing that the genetic lottery will not have treated all groups the same does not mean that we are duty bound to treat such groups differently. The salient Aristotelian principle of treating like things alike assumes that we have already agreed upon what things are worthy of consideration. Those things that determine humanness and standing are most of all socially determined and fixed by circumstances of personal history and socioeconomic factors. They are least of all those things that are genetic. Even where there are genetic factors at play, as is likely to be true for manic–depressive psychosis, policies that recognize the human needs of such individuals are of necessity "gene blind" as well as color blind. For almost every infirmity that has a genetic basis, there is a "phenocopy" that is solely the result of environmental forces. So here, treating like things alike means ignoring the causal factors and treating the person. For this reason, social policies directed against genetic impairments—real or predicted by the human genome's revelations—are almost always secondary to social policies directed against the environmental causes of human injustice. In any case, deciding how to incorporate new genetic data into social policy and how to compensate people with important genetic differences will thus be a daunting task. Just how we will incorporate the traditional American values of justice and fair play into the genetic lottery is perhaps the largest, long-term challenge posed by the genome project. How we do so will be a measure of our humanity as well as our science.

NOTES

1. See especially Diana Brahams, "Human Genetic Information: The Legal Implications," *Human Genetic Information: Science, Law, and Ethics* (Chichester, U.K.: John Wiley & Sons, 1990), *Ciba Foundation Symposium* 149 (1990): 111–132.

2. U.S. Department of Health and Human Services, *The Human Genome Project: New Tools for Tomorrow's Health Research* (1991), 3.

3. Ibid., 3–4.

4. See C. Wills, *Exons, Introns, and Talking Genes: The Science Behind the Human Genome Project* (New York: Basic Books, 1991).

5. Ibid., 3.

6. See R. C. Lewontin and D. L. Hartl, "Population Genetics in Forensic DNA Typing," *Science* 295 (1991): 1745–1750.

7. A. E. Mourant, *The Distribution of the Human Blood Groups* (Oxford, U.K.: Blackwell, 1954).

8. See Marc Lappé, "Ethical Issues in Screening for Chronic Lung Disease," *Journal of Occupational Medicine* 30(1988): 493–501.

9. R. C. Lewontin and D. L. Hartl, "Response," *Science* 255 (1992): 1054–1055.

10. S. S. Deeb, R. A. Failor, B. G. Brown, J. D. Brunzell, A. G. Motulsky et al., "Association of Apolipoprotein B Gene Variants with Plasma apoB and Low Density Lipoprotein (LDL) Cholesterol Levels," *Human Genetics* 88(1992): 463–470.

11. See Marc Lappé, *Genetic Politics* (New York: Simon and Schuster, 1987).

12. B. P. Dohernwend, I. Levav, P. E. Shrout, et al., "Socioeconomic Status and Psychiatric Disorders: The Causation–Selection Issues," *Science* 255 (1992): 946–951.

13. See Constance Holden, "Depression: The News Isn't Depressing," *Science* 254 (1991): 1451–1453.

14. David W. E. Smith, "Variability in Life Span Functional Capacity," in A. D. Woodhead, M. A. Bender, and R. C. Leonard, *Phenotypic Variation in Populations, Basic Life Sciences,* vol. 43 (New York: Plenum Press, 1988), 172–180.

15. See John Rawls, *A Theory of Justice* (Cambridge, MA: Harvard University Press, 1971).

16. "The Declaration of Inuyama and Reports of the Working Groups," *Human Gene Therapy* 21 (1991): 123–129.

17. See Stephen L. Brown, "Differential Susceptibility: Implications for Epidemiology, Risk Assessment, and Public Policy," in Woodhead et al., *Phenotypic Variation in Populations,* 255–270.

18. Lappé, "Ethical Issues."

19. See K. Honda et al., "HLA and silicosis in Japan," *New England Journal of Medicine* 319 (1988): 1610

NOTES ON CONTRIBUTORS

Lori B. Andrews is a graduate of Yale Law School and is currently a Research Fellow at the American Bar Foundation and a Senior Scholar at the Center for Clinical Medical Ethics at the University of Chicago. She has taught health law at the University of Chicago School of Law and at the University of Chicago Business School. She has written extensively on genetics, reproductive technologies, and other aspects of medical law. She has been an advisor to various federal health and scientific agencies. She is co-chair of the American Bar Association Task Force on Reproductive and Genetic Technologies.

George J. Annas is Edward R. Utley Professor of Law and Medicine at the Boston University Schools of Medicine and Public Health. He is also the Director of the Law, Medicine, and Ethics Program at Boston University School of Public Health. He is the author of more than 200 articles and the author or editor of a number of books on the rights of patients, genetics and the law, informed consent, the rights of health care professionals, reproductive genetics, and most recently, *The Nazi Doctors and the Nuremberg Code: Human Rights in Human Experimentation* (Oxford, 1992).

Arthur Caplan is Director of the Center for Biomedical Ethics, as well as professor of philosophy and professor of surgery at the University of Minnesota. He is the author or editor of fifteen books, including *If I Were a Rich Man I Could Buy a Pancreas* (Indiana, 1992), *Which Babies Shall Live?* (Humana, 1985), *The Sociobiology Debate* (Harper & Row, 1978), *Concepts of Health and Disease* (Addison-Wesley, 1981), and *In Search of Equity* (Plenum, 1983). He has written widely in the fields of philosophy, medicine, and the biological sciences; is a frequent commentator in the media; and has served as a consultant to a wide range of governmental agencies.

Norman Daniels, Professor and Chair of the Tufts University Philosophy Department, has written widely in the philosophy of science, ethics, political and social philosophy, and medical ethics. His most recent books include *Just Health Care* (Cambridge, 1985) and *Am I My Parents' Keeper: An Essay on Justice between the Young and the Old* (Oxford, 1988). He is currently receiving support from the National Endowment for the Humanities and the National Library of Medicine to write a book on justice and AIDS policy choices.

Leonard M. Fleck is an Associate Professor in the Philosophy Department and Center for Humanities in the Life Sciences at Michigan State University. He has published over thirty-five articles and book chapters that address a range of issues connected with justice and health care policy. He is the director of a statewide community education project in Michigan titled "Just Caring: Conflicting Rights, Uncertain Responsibilities," which is exploring democratic decision-making approaches to health care rationing. He continues to work on a book titled *Pricing Human Life: Moral and Public Policy Dilemmas.*

Daniel J. Kevles is the Koepfli Professor of the Humanities at the California Institute of Technology, where he heads the Program on Science, Ethics, and Public Policy. He is the coeditor, with Leroy Hood, of *The Code of Codes: Scientific and Social Issues in the Human Genome Project* (Harvard, 1992) and is currently completing a book on the essence and ownership of life.

Marc A. Lappé is Professor of Health Policy and Ethics in the Department of Medical Education at the University of Illinois College of Medicine at Chicago. He has had a broad background straddling fields in science, ethics, and health policy, having held positions at the University of California and at the Hastings Center, as well as in various state and federal agencies. He has written more than 100 publications, including five books and several chapters in public health, policy, and toxicology texts. His most recent book is *Chemical Deception* (Sierra Club Books, 1991), which examines myths about toxic substances.

Timothy F. Murphy is Assistant Professor of Philosophy in the Biomedical Sciences, Department of Medical Education, at the University of Illinois College of Medicine at Chicago. He is the coeditor, with Suzanne Poirier, of *Writing AIDS: Gay Literature, Language, and Analysis* (Columbia, 1993), the editor of *Gay Ethics: Outing, Civil Rights, and the Meaning of Science* (Haworth Press, 1994), and the author of a forthcoming book, *Ethics in an Epidemic: AIDS, Morality, and Culture* (California, 1994).

Robert J. Pokorski is Vice President, Medical Research, of North American Reassurance. He directs medical research and development and is responsible for developing underwriting guidelines that reflect recent trends in medical care and longevity. He is a member of the American Council of Life

Insurance Medical Section Genetic Testing Committee, having formerly served as chairman of that committee. He is also a member of the Association of Life Insurance Medical Directors of America. Dr. Pokorski earned his medical degree at Creighton University, is certified by the American Board of Internal Medicine and the Board of Insurance Medicine, and is a fellow of the American College of Physicians.

Index

Designer:	U.C. Press Staff
Compositor:	Impressions
Text:	11/13 Baskerville
Display:	Baskerville
Printer:	Edwards Bros.
Binder:	Edwards Bros.